# the brilliant
# carbs
# counter

# the brilliant
# carbs
# counter

carolyn humphries

## foulsham
LONDON • NEW YORK • TORONTO • SYDNEY

# foulsham

Capital Point, 33 Bath Road, Slough, Berkshire, SL1 3UF, England

Foulsham books can be found in all good bookshops and direct from www.foulsham.com

ISBN: 978-0-572-03687-4

A CIP record for this book is available from the British Library.

Cover photograph © Superstock

Printed in Great Britain by Thomson Litho, East Kilbride

# Contents

# Introduction

E ven dieters of 50 years ago would agree that if you cut out bread, potatoes, other starches and sugar – which are high in calories – you'll lose weight. But it's the science behind the dieting that's changed. It's now believed that as your body normally converts carbohydrates into glucose to use as energy, if you cut down drastically on carbohydrates your body has to burn body fat for energy instead. You also need to eat more fats and proteins, so instead of a limp lettuce leaf, you can enjoy a surprisingly indulgent eating plan, like tucking in to a huge steak, topping your salad with a dollop of mayonnaise and even having cream in your coffee! If you follow the concept properly, you'll lose weight rapidly at first, then more slowly until you can maintain a new, slimmer you for life.

This book gives you all the basic low-down you need to understand a low-carbohydrate diet plus a really comprehensive, easy-reference carbohydrates counter, which gives you not only the grams of carbohydrates in just about any food you want to eat but also the calories, protein, fat and fibre content too.

You should, however, research several different low-carb diets. They all vary slightly, even though the basic concepts are the same. Some may suit you better than others.

# The Low-carbohydrate, High-protein Diet

A low-carbohydrate/high-protein diet is very different from a low-calorie one. On a low-calorie reducing diet, you have to eat far fewer calories than your body needs each day for energy so the body burns stored body fat for fuel instead. It can also use lean muscle tissue, so you will reduce in size as well as lose weight. But the loss of muscle tissue can cause a reduction in the rate of your metabolism, which means that your rate of weight loss will drop. That is the moment at which you can become demoralised and stop the low-calorie intake. You will then rapidly revert to your former size – or bigger (and flabbier) – because you will simply re-store fat very quickly.

On a low-carbohydrate/high-protein diet, you introduce a new way of eating for life. You re-educate your body to eating differently long term. As I said, you seriously restrict carbohydrates at first, gradually re-introducing some, on a limited basis, in phases. You also eat more pure fats and proteins, so the body doesn't use muscle tissue for energy, just fat. You can lose and sustain your weight loss but won't necessarily become thin with a reduced rate of metabolism. This kind of diet is not designed as a 'quick fix' solution (although many famous people go on the first stage of the diet from time to time to lose weight rapidly for a particular part or to look svelt for a special occasion). If you do as they do, your body will fluctuate from balloon to stick – very depressing and not healthy! If you follow your chosen regime and stick to it – not just selected parts of it – you should be able to reduce weight and stay slimmer and healthier.

## How does a low-carbohydrate/high-protein diet work?

This is a basic introduction to this type of diet. To understand it fully, you should read a few different low-carbohydrate diet books.

1. The body breaks down carbohydrates into glucose to use as energy. If people eat more carbohydrates than their body burns, they are stored in the body as fat.

2. As long as the body has enough carbohydrates to convert to glucose for energy, it won't burn up any body fat. But if the body doesn't have enough glucose in the body (that is, by not eating enough carbohydrates) the body is forced to burn body fat for energy instead. It would also burn protein for energy, thus reducing muscle tissue, which is why you increase your protein intake on this type of diet to prevent that from happening.

3. When you eat carbohydrates, the pancreas produces insulin to help the body absorb the glucose for energy. The more starch and sugar you eat, the more insulin is produced. Insulin also helps the body to store any unused glucose as fat. So when you severely restrict carbohydrates, the body no longer makes loads of insulin and so does not make or store body fat.

4. When the body is starved of carbohydrates for energy, the liver produces ketones from fatty acids for energy instead. Any excess ketones are passed out of the body in the urine so are not stored as fat. This process is called ketosis and is of prime importance in some – but not all – low-carbohydrate diets. For the pros and cons of ketosis, see opposite.

5. Once your body is free from large quantities of carbohydrates, blood sugar levels should remain constant, so you are unlikely to have cravings for sugar or serious hunger pangs. But the body does need a small amount of glucose for some vital functions. This is achieved by either eating a few carbohydrates or, when necessary, the liver can process proteins and turn them into sugar.

## The pros and cons of ketosis

When your body produces ketones from fat for energy, they cannot be turned back into fat, so any unused ones are excreted from the body rather than stored as fat. Ketosis is a natural function – the back-up system that starts to operate when the body does not have enough glucose to convert to energy. But the downside is that the process causes severe bad breath and a metallic taste in the mouth, which many find very unpleasant (and antisocial).

Some diets recommend that you test your urine for ketones as often as twice a day with a special kit normally used by diabetics – a nuisance, to say the least! There is some controversy as to whether ketosis is dangerous in the long term, so do not stay on the first part of the diet for more than two weeks.

Note that ketosis is NOT Ketoacidosis, a dangerous condition that occurs in people with diabetes when their blood pH becomes acutely acidic and their blood sugar levels soar because they either are not producing insulin or are not responding to it so can't process sugar for energy. The body then produces ketones for fuel instead.

# A Healthy Lifestyle

The principle of a low-carbohydrate diet is that instead of your body converting carbohydrates to glucose for energy, it has to burn fat instead. Now, cutting them down drastically for a short time for quick weight loss is okay but you cannot and must not maintain this regime for too long or you will become lethargic and ill. Your body needs nutrients from all the food groups to maintain health and vitality. That is why there are stages on a low-carbohydrate diet to make sure that you do not lack vital goodness for health in the long term. In the long term, your body must have the right balance of the following food types.

## Proteins

These are used by the body for growth and repair and, when necessary, for energy. The best sources are fish, lean meat, poultry, dairy products, eggs, soya proteins such as tofu, and Quorn (made from a fungus). Pulses (dried peas, beans and lentils) are also good sources of protein but as they are also high in carbohydrates, they will have to be avoided at least until the latter stages of this diet (and then only eaten in moderation). As you are going to be on a low-carbohydrate diet, you will be eating more proteins (and fats) than usual.

## Carbohydrates

There are two types of carbohydrates. Complex carbo-hydrates are all the starchy foods like bread (all types), pasta, rice, cereals (including breakfast cereals) and starchy vegetables like potatoes. Simple carbohydrates are sugars and include those naturally found in foods – like fructose in fruit and lactose in milk – as well as refined sugars used in cakes, biscuits (cookies) and sweets (candies).

Nutritionally, the starchy ones and the natural sugars in milk, fruit, etc., are usually considered the 'good' foods and are used solely for energy. However, when on a weight-reducing low-carbohydrate plan, these are the foods to reduce drastically in the first phase of the diet, then to re-introduce slowly, without eating to excess. Refined sugars are to be avoided.

## Fats

These can also be converted by the body into energy when carbohydrates are limited, and are also used for warmth. They are found naturally in foods high in protein such as dairy products, meat, fish, poultry, nuts and seeds, and also in some fruits such as olives and avocados (which makes these a positive bonus on the low-carbohydrate plan).

## Fibre

This is vital for healthy body functioning. One of the main problems with a low-carbohydrate diet is that it can be low in fibre. To compensate for this, eat lots of dark green vegetables and lots of nuts and seeds as soon as you are allowed. Drink plenty of water and take plenty of exercise, too, to help prevent constipation. When, later, you are able to have potatoes and fruit, like apples, eat the skin as well. You can bake scrubbed potato peelings in a hot oven for about 20 minutes until crisp and golden, then season them with salt and pepper for a delicious, much lower-carb-than-whole-potato snack (only 7g carbohydrates per medium potato). See also watch points, page 24.

## Drinks

Make sure you drink plenty of water from the tap, or filtered, mineral or no-calorie flavoured waters, according to your preference. Some low-carbohydrate diets recommend you avoid caffeine (tea, coffee, hot chocolate, cola, etc.) because it may trigger insulin production, which would impair weight loss (see page 8). Others leave it up to you. I suggest that you drink weak black (or with cream, not milk) tea or coffee at first or, if in doubt, choose caffeine-free tea or coffee, or have herb tea. I would stress, though, that coffee and cocoa contain small amounts of carbohydrates, so you have to include them in your counting; tea has none.

You may also have no-carbohydrate (diet) soft drinks, carbohydrate-free clear soup and pure lemon or lime juice with water (artificially sweetened, if necessary). There are traces of carbohydrates in lemons and limes but not as much as in other fruit juices.

Do not drink milk, sweet pure juices or soft drinks sweetened with sugar.

Alcohol is not recommended on some low-carbohydrate diets; others allow it in moderation. Dry wines and spirits have only a trace of carbohydrates but avoid beers, sweet and fortified wines and liqueurs. Remember, though, that alcohol is easily burned by your body for energy, so will be used before any fat. If you enjoy a drink, have one – but not too many! Always have no-calorie mixers with spirits and drink plenty of water before and after. Also, ideally, eat foods high in protein when drinking alcohol.

## Vitamins and minerals

A balanced diet of fresh foods should contain sufficient vitamins and minerals for general health and well-being. The following chart will help you to identify which foods contain which nutrients so you can try to get a good balance.

Because you are going to reduce the amount of carbohydrates you eat, you may also be restricting some vital nutrients. Many vitamins and minerals, for example, are found in fruits and vegetables, whether fresh, frozen or canned in water or natural juice with no added sugar (and, ideally, no added salt). It is generally recommended that you eat at least five portions of these a day. Make sure, while on the initial quick-weight-loss part of the diet, that you eat as many as you can of the fruits and vegetables that are allowed to try to get as many of these important nutrients into your diet as possible to compensate for the ones you cannot have.

As you progress through the plan, you will be able to introduce more vegetable variety and some fruit as well, which makes it easier to maintain your vitamin and mineral intake.

For information, I have also included in the chart the foods that contain the relevant nutrient but are high in carbohydrates.

If you are on a low-carbohydrate diet, you may become deficient in some vital nutrients, especially in the early quick-weight-loss phase. Some dieticians have their own recommendations about specific supplement formulas, but I recommend that you take a good-quality multi-vitamin and mineral supplement that includes calcium, as well as eating a variety of the foods you can eat from the list overleaf. Make sure that it contains no sugar or starch. I do not recommend that you take other individual supplements as you can overdose, which can be as harmful to your health as a deficiency.

| Vitamin | Important for | Vitamin-rich foods |
| --- | --- | --- |
| Vitamin A | Colour and night vision; healthy skin and mucous membranes | Liver, butter, eggs, whole milk products (e.g. full-fat cheeses), fish liver oils, green, orange and red vegetables, fortified margarines |
| B Vitamin complex | | |
| Thiamin ($B_1$) | Conversion of carbohydrates to energy; function of the central nervous system | Cheese, meat, yeast extract *High-carb*: milk and other milk products, bread and other cereals, potatoes |
| Riboflavin ($B_2$) | Conversion of carbohydrates, fats and proteins to energy; healthy skin and eyes | Eggs, cheese, meat (especially offal), poultry, yeast extract, vegetables *High-carb*: milk and other milk products, fortified breakfast cereals |
| Niacin (Nicotinic acid) | Conversion of carbohydrates, fats and proteins to energy | Meat and meat products, poultry, fish *High-carb*: fortified breakfast cereals, bread, potatoes |
| Vitamin $B_6$ | Conversion of proteins, fats and carbohydrates to energy; function of the central nervous system | Meat, poultry, vegetables *High-carb*: fruit, potatoes, cereals, pulses (dried peas, beans and lentils) |

| Vitamin | Important for | Vitamin-rich foods |
|---|---|---|
| Vitamin B$_{12}$ | Function of the central nervous system; production of red blood cells; metabolism of DNA and RNA; growth | Meat and meat products (especially liver), cheese, eggs, fish, yeast extract<br>*High-carb:* milk, fortified breakfast cereals |
| Folic acid | Function of the central nervous system; production of red blood cells; synthesis of DNA | Offal, green leafy vegetables (especially raw ones)<br>*High-carb:* oranges, wholegrain cereals |
| Pantothenic acid | Conversion of fats and proteins to energy | Offal, fresh vegetables, peanuts<br>*High-carb:* pulses (dried peas, beans, lentils), fortified breakfast cereals |
| Biotin | Conversion of fats and proteins to energy | Cheese, vegetables, fish, egg yolk, offal<br>*High-carb:* milk and other milk products, fruit, cereals |
| Vitamin C | Production of collagen for connective tissue, blood vessels and capillaries; support of the immune system and healing; absorption of iron; lipid metabolism; detoxification (for alcohol and drugs) | Vegetables (especially green vegetables, (bell) peppers)<br>*High-carb:* potatoes, pure fruit juices, fruit (especially blackcurrants, strawberries, kiwis and citrus) |

| Vitamin | Important for | Vitamin-rich foods |
|---|---|---|
| Vitamin D | Growth and maintenance of healthy teeth and bones; absorption of calcium | Sunshine, butter, eggs, oily fish, fortified margarines<br>High-carb: fortified breakfast cereals |
| Vitamin E | Protection of cell membranes; prevention of lipid damage from oxidation | Eggs, dark leafy vegetables, vegetable oils<br>High-carb: wholegrain cereals |
| Vitamin K | Metabolism of energy; blood clotting | Vegetables, especially brassicas (cabbage, cauliflower etc.) and spinach |
| Essential fatty acids<br>Linoleic acid (Omega-3)<br>Linolenic acid (Omega-6)<br>Oleic acid | General good health | Oily fish, vegetable seeds and seed oils, polyunsaturated margarines, olive oil, nuts and nut oils |

| Mineral | Important for | Mineral-rich foods |
|---------|---------------|--------------------|
| Calcium | Healthy growth and development of bones and teeth; release of hormones in the body | Canned fish (especially the bones), green vegetables *High-carb:* milk and milk products, bread |
| Chromium | Activating insulin which controls the use of glucose in the body | Most foods, particularly vegetables *High-carb:* particularly wholegrain cereals |
| Copper | Production of enzymes, especially those involved with the blood and bones and the immune system; aiding neurotransmission; respiration of cells | Vegetables, meat, oysters, nuts *High-carb:* wholegrain cereals |
| Fluorine | Prevention of tooth decay | Fish, water, tea |
| Iodine | Regulation of many body processes, via the thyroid hormones | Meat, fish, eggs, cheese, iodised salt *High-carb:* milk and other milk products |
| Iron | Formation of red blood cells; transportation and transfer of oxygen; metabolism of drugs | Meat (especially offal), vegetables *High-carb:* potatoes, bread and cereal products |

| Mineral | Important for | Mineral-rich foods |
|---|---|---|
| Magnesium | Muscle tone; enzyme activation, especially to break down proteins | Vegetables, nuts<br>High-carb: milk, bread and cereal products, potatoes |
| Manganese | Maintenance of healthy cells; activation of enzymes; helping the utilisation of calcium and potassium | Nuts, tea<br>High-carb: wholegrain cereals |
| Molybdenum | Production of many enzymes, especially for the formation of uric acid; metabolism of DNA | Most foods, particularly vegetables<br>High-carb: particularly pulses (dried peas, beans and lentils) |
| Phosphorus | Production of all cells; aiding storage of energy, membrane function, growth and reproduction | Meat and meat products, cheese, cream<br>High-carb: milk and other milk products, bread and cereal products |
| Potassium | Maintenance of water levels in the body | Vegetables, meat<br>High-carb: milk, fruit and pure fruit juices |
| Selenium | Production of an enzyme in red blood cells; protection of membranes | Fish, cheese, eggs, meat (especially offal)<br>High-carb: milk, cereals |
| Sodium and chlorine | Maintenance of water levels in the body | Meat products, cooking and table salt<br>High-carb: milk, bread and cereal products |

| Mineral | Important for | Mineral-rich foods |
| --- | --- | --- |
| Zinc | Metabolism of bones; release of Vitamin A and insulin; activation of enzymes; growth; support of the immune system; taste | Meat and meat products, cheese<br>*High-carb*: milk and other milk products, bread and cereal products |

## Regular exercise

Exercise is vital for stimulating the metabolism. An active body is more likely to be a healthy body. One mad burst a week at the gym isn't a good idea. You need to go more frequently to reap the benefit, if you like that sort of thing. But there are plenty of ways to get regular exercise without jogging or work-outs.

- Walk briskly instead of wandering along and certainly walk instead of using the car or public transport whenever possible.

- If you take the bus, get off a stop before your usual one and walk the last part of the journey.

- Ride a bike if you have one.

- Use the stairs instead of lifts or escalators.

- Take up a recreational sport like tennis or swimming, or another activity like a dance class or gardening.

- Bending and stretching exercises will also help to tone your muscles but you must do them properly or you can cause yourself damage. Seek advice before you start. If you are going to do some at home, make them a regular part of your daily routine, perhaps as soon as you get out of bed or before you have your shower or bath in the morning or evening. If you don't, the novelty will wear off after a few days and you won't persevere.

# The Stages of the Low-carbohydrate Diet

There are several variations on the low-carb diet. The most comprehensive has four phases; others have fewer phases. The different diets do vary slightly in what they allow, so this should be treated as a general guide only.

### Phase one: the quick-weight-loss phase

This is often called the induction phase. I recommend you do not go on this part of the diet for more than two weeks as many nutrients are severely restricted.

- During the first phase you cut out most carbohydrates. The amount will depend on which diet you follow. You may be allowed as little as 20 g a day (when you will definitely produce lots of ketones and suffer the side-effects (see page 9)), or as much as 120 g a day, 40 per cent of the normal recommended amount (300 g). Only eat foods from those allowed for this phase (see the list below).

- Make sure you eat as many permitted salads and vegetables as you can within the amount of carbohydrates allowed on your diet. It is best to have the ones lowest in carbohydrates in larger quantities, particularly dark green ones and celery as they have the most fibre.

- You can eat as much pure protein and fat as you need to fill you up.

- Only eat when you are hungry and eat just enough to satisfy you. Don't eat for the sake of it. Do not eat forbidden foods at all – not even a tiny amount – or the diet won't work.

- Use the carbohydrates counter to check everything you are eating. That way you will be able to stick rigorously to the diet. I have rounded up each food to the nearest gramme, so you know you will never be over your limit. It also prevents having to do difficult sums with decimal points!

- Beware of foods with just a trace of carbohydrates in them. This means they have less than 0.5 g of carbohydrates per portion. If you eat lots of them, however, you could increase your carbohydrate intake by a gram or two (which is only vital on the early stages of the extremely low-carb diets).

## Foods you are allowed

### Eat as much as you like of:

- All plain cooked meat and poultry, including beef, pork, lamb, veal, bacon, pure gammon ham (no crumb coating or processed pork with additives), rabbit, venison, chicken, turkey, duck, goose, pheasant, quail, grouse and other game. Note that some offal, like liver is extremely nutritious but does have a small amount of carbohydrates, so make sure you include them in your calculations.

- All plain cooked fish and shellfish, such as cod, haddock, sole, tuna, salmon, sardines, mackerel, prawns (shrimp), crabmeat (not dressed crab as it contains breadcrumbs), lobster, oysters, mussels, clams, squid. Note that some shellfish naturally contain small amounts of carbohydrates; they will need to be included in your calculations.

- All hard and fresh cheeses, such as Cheddar, Edam, Stilton, Dolcelatte, Mozzarella, Camembert, goats' and sheep's cheeses. Note that cheeses have small amounts of carbohydrates in them, so if eating a lot, remember to add them to your calculations. Whey cheeses such as Ricotta are not allowed.

- Pure fats, such as butter, olive, seed and vegetable oils, cream (unsweetened fresh, soured (dairy sour) and crème fraîche, but beware 'light' cream substitutes). Note that all creams contain small amounts of carbohydrates, so, if eating a lot, remember to include them in your calculation. Also note that some diets forbid margarine.

- Eggs (cooked by any method).

## Eat the quantities allowed in your diet of:

- Vegetables with less than 10g carbohydrates per portion: artichokes, asparagus, aubergine (eggplant), bamboo shoots, bean sprouts, broccoli, Brussels sprouts, all types of cabbage, carrots, cauliflower, celeriac (celery root), courgettes (zucchini), French (green) or runner beans, kale, kohlrabi, leeks, mangetout (snow peas), all types of mushrooms, okra, onions, pak choi, palm hearts, pumpkin, spinach, spring (collard) greens, swede (rutabaga), swiss chard, turnip, water chestnuts. You may also eat rhubarb (with artificial sweetener), which is a vegetable.

- Fruit (the only ones you are allowed now): avocado, olives, tomatoes.

- Salad stuffs: celery, chicory (Belgian endive), cucumber, fennel, fresh herbs, all types of red and green lettuce, (bell) peppers, radishes, rocket, sorrel, watercress.

- Spices: all types provided there is no starchy filler of sugar in the mix.

**Foods you are not allowed**
- Any processed meat, poultry or fish products, such as sausages, fish fingers, southern fried chicken, pâtés.

- Any dairy products except cheese, cream and butter.

- Any fruit except the three listed above.

- Any starchy foods like bread, potatoes, pasta, rice or other grains.

- Any sugar or sweetened foods (other than with artificial sweetener).

## Watch points

**Feeling strange:** It is possible that to start with you may feel light-headed early on because of the lack of starchy fillers. If so, nibble a small finger of hard cheese. It has only a tiny amount of carbohydrates but will stop that dizzy feeling. Alternatively you could feel nauseous because of the change in your protein and fat intake. I suggest sipping sparkling water, plain or flavoured with pure lemon or lime juice. If you have a sweet tooth, an artificially sweetened flavoured seltzer is a good idea. Alternatively, sip mint tea.

**Upset tummy:** It is quite common for people to get diarrhoea when they first embark on a low-carb diet. It happens particularly if the person is not used to eating lots of raw salad stuffs. If you have wind as well, try lightly cooking vegetables and dressing them with oil and vinegar instead of having raw salads. It is important to chew all raw veggies thoroughly because otherwise they are difficult to digest.

Another cause can be the added fat in your diet. If you were on a low-fat regime before, the added oils, butter and cream could be enough to cause your upset tummy. Provided you are not in pain, the problem should right itself.

If you are using a lot of artificial sweeteners, these may be causing the problem, either because they contain sorbitol, which has a laxative effect, or because they contain maltodextrin as a bulky filler to make the product more like ordinary sugar. This, too, can cause diarrhoea in some people.

If you have serious bloating, flatulence and cramp-like pains, you may have a food intolerance or even irritable bowel syndrome. You should seek medical advice before continuing with the diet.

## Phase two: the ongoing weight-loss phase

At this stage, you start gradually to build up your carbohydrates, increasing your carbohydrates slightly so you still lose 500 g–1 kg/1–2 lb per week. Some plans suggest you go up in 5 g of carb increments per week. If you increase too quickly, you'll plateau (see pages 27–8) or start to increase weight again. If you keep it too low, ketosis will start, if it hasn't already, which you may or may not want. If you are losing weight rapidly, increase the carbohydrates by a few grams. Too rapid a weight loss after the initial loss is not good in the long term. It must be a gradual process.

**Foods you are allowed**

You can, of course, increase the amount of vegetables already allowed (thus slightly increasing your carbohydrate allowance) but you can now add any of the following as well:

- Nuts and seeds (low in carbs but high in fibre).
- Low-carb soft fruits: raspberries, strawberries, blackberries, cherries and physalis.

## Watch points

**Ketosis:** Extreme low-carb diets encourage you to persevere with the ketosis (the bad breath and metallic taste in the mouth etc., from the production of ketones in the body) but many health professionals suggest it may be dangerous and think it should be toned down (even if it means losing weight slightly less quickly). You can do this by eating a small amount of slightly higher-carbohydrate foods like carrots, red (bell) peppers or even an apple or pear which, although 'off limits' on the strict low-carb regime, are preferable to having refined sugar and are not as high in carbohydrates as starchy foods like potatoes, rice or bread.

**Excessive proteins:** There is a possible danger, in the long term, of having too much protein on a regular basis. It can put a strain on the kidneys and the liver. It is therefore vital that you keep increasing the vegetables and fruits you are allowed, not piling on even more protein.

**Low fibre:** The lack of fibre on a low-carb diet can cause problems with digestion. As stressed already, it is very important to drink plenty of water and eat lots of nuts and seeds, and as many fruit and vegetables as you are allowed. If you should suffer from constipation, try buying flax meal or seeds to sprinkle on your food, according to the directions. Alternatively, an extra tablespoon of olive oil a day (maybe on your salad) can help. If not, you can buy natural health preparations from your health food shop, which should help.

## Phase three: the pre-maintenance phase

This is the when-you're-almost-there-adding-extras phase. Although you may be anxious to keep up a rapid weight loss, try not to be too impatient; if you lose weight too quickly it is not healthy and the weight is far less likely to remain off in the long term. That is why you can now include a 'treat' once or twice a week, such as a glass of wine (if that wasn't allowed before!), a jacket potato, a peach or a slice of wholemeal bread. By this stage you should be feeling really fit and healthy.

However, this is often the trickiest phase because, as you are able to indulge in a few extra carbs, it is easy to go over the top. Also, by adding these extra carbohydrates, your appetite will no longer be suppressed by ketone production, so you may start to feel hungrier than you did before, which could lead to overeating. Providing you don't overdo things, you will reach your goal in a few weeks and can then, ideally, set about maintaining the diet for the rest of your life.

## Watch points

**The problem of the plateau:** Many people will reach an impasse at this point. Providing you are not actually gaining weight, your carbohydrate levels are about right. If you are putting it on again, cut back on the carbs. Don't worry until the plateau has continued for more than three or four weeks. Your body may just be 'regrouping' so, if you don't give up the regime, you will begin to lose weight again. Also, check your measurements. If you've lost in size all you wanted, you may already have reached your goal, even if it is a couple of kilos/pounds heavier than you'd originally planned. If, however, you still have a little bit to lose, there are ways to try and kick-start the diet.

- You could have a day or two of fruit only BUT for no more than two days.

- Or go on a properly balanced calorie-controlled phase for a week or two, then go back to the low-carb regime (you can use this book to give you the calorie counts of everything you eat, but stick to 1,000–1,200 calories per day for a woman, 1,200–1,500 for a man). At the end of two weeks, go back to phase two of the low-carb diet then continue as before.

- You may just be consuming lots of hidden carbohydrates. See page 33 for more information and make sure you cut them out so you get back to the carb level you really want.

One thing you must not do is stay on the low-carb diet but reduce the amount of protein and fats you are eating. If you do that you won't be getting enough nutrients and you will slow your metabolism right down so you don't lose at all.

**Reverting to bad old ways:** Because you can now have 'treats' it is very easy to think 'an extra bar of chocolate won't hurt'. On its own, it probably won't. The trouble is, before you know it you will keep telling yourself all the time that 'the odd this and that doesn't matter' and you'll have started eating biscuits, chocolates, sweets, sugary puds – the lot! Having trained your body so well for so long, you shouldn't throw it all away now. Remember, treats really should be treats and only a couple of times a week!

## Phase four: the maintenance phase

This is also known as the diet-for-life phase. Now you have reached your goal. You are the desired weight/size you want to be. Having got here, you have already gone through the gradual inclusion of carbohydrate 'treats' so now you can gradually include any fruit and vegetables you like and whole grains like oats, wheat, barley, millet, wholemeal pasta or brown rice, etc. Ideally, avoid processed carbohydrates, like white bread, white rice, etc., and it is recommended that you only have sugary foods as very special treats. They can undo all the good work very quickly! You must still keep a record of the amount of carbs you are eating, so you will know exactly what level will keep your weight constant.

The important thing is to weigh yourself regularly. If you find you are gaining weight, you must cut back on the carbohydrates until you find the level that means you can sustain your ideal weight. So, for instance, you may find that at 120 g of carbohydrates a day, you can keep your weight exactly the same, but if it rises to 150 g a day, you start to put on weight. The amount of carbohydrates people can tolerate varies enormously.

## Watch points

**Overeating:** Doctors and scientists don't seem to be able to agree on whether this kind of diet is good for you in the long term. If you want to err on the side of caution, I suggest the following approach. When you are eating a reasonable quantity of carbohydrates, make sure you don't eat even more proteins and fats too. If you do, you will be consuming too much food in undesirable quantities. So, once you've reached your desired weight, it is a good idea to watch calories as well as carbohydrates and work towards a balance

29

of lots of fruit and vegetables, rather less proteins and fats; a reasonable amount of starchy carbohydrates and very little added sugar, allowing no more than 2,000 calories a day for a woman, 2,500 calories a day for a man.

# Planning Your Diet

It is important before you embark on any reducing diet that you check with your doctor that you are basically fit and healthy. If, for instance, you are already on a low-fat regime or a low-cholesterol diet for medical reasons, it may not be suitable for you to go on a low-carb diet. If you are diabetic, you must not go on this without the agreement of your doctor. You would have to be closely monitored and your blood sugar level must be kept low and stable. Never 'go it alone'!

## Identify how much you have to lose

You know in your heart when you are overweight. Your clothes don't hang properly, they feel tight or you have to buy a larger size than you did before. If you look at yourself without clothes, you see rolls of flab where, maybe, you were once firm or at least only gently curving. Your stomach appears swollen even if you try hard to draw it in, you have more than one chin and you appear puffy. Some of you will only need to trim down a little; others will have a lot more to lose.

Overleaf is a chart, based on UK government statistics, which shows you how much you should weigh according to your height. It depends on your bone structure as to whether you will be at the lower end of the scale or higher up. The important thing is to be within the limits of ideal weight.

Weigh yourself first thing in the morning, preferably without clothes. (If you weigh with light clothes on, make sure each time that you have on similar clothes.) Look where you are on the scale, then work out how much weight you need to lose. Once you've made that calculation, weigh regularly, but not every day. I do it once a week, but some people prefer to weigh more frequently, even if their weight fluctuates (as it will). Remember that on a low-carb diet, you may lose weight but not so many inches.

Also record your body measurements before you start your diet. Measure your chest/bust, waist and hips. Also make a note of your upper arm measurement, your thighs, calves and neck. That way, when you are well into your diet you will be able to check how much body mass you've lost even if your weight loss slows down considerably. When you replace fat with lean muscle tissue, you will be smaller in size even if you aren't still losing weight.

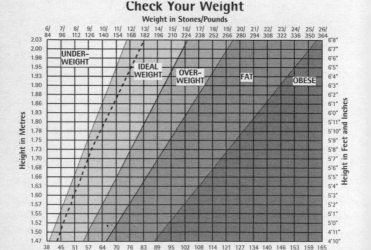

**Check Your Weight**

# Hidden Carbohydrates

We all know that carbohydrates are starchy foods like bread, pasta, rice and potatoes and that sugars are sweet things like fruit, cakes, chocolate, biscuits, sweets (candies) and ice cream, but there are lots of other foods that are surprising sources too. Most importantly be wary of any food that claims to be 'low fat' or 'light': they will nearly always have added starches or sugars to compensate for the reduced amount of fat!

Always read the labels to make informed choices (and check in this book). As I have mentioned before, in the book if an item has a trace of carbohydrates, it means it has less than 0.5 g carbohydrates per serving. But if you have several portions, you could be increasing your carbs by another gram or two, so bear this in mind when calculating on the first phase of your diet, especially if it is one which only allows you a tiny amount of carbohydrates.

## Meats, seafood and poultry

Delicatessen meats; processed meat products, like sausages, frankfurters, pâtés, corned beef and potted meats; crab sticks and other imitation fish products; fish fingers and pastes; canned fish in sauce; shaped chicken and turkey fingers/ drumsticks and so on. Note too that, as I've said before, some offal and fish contain small amounts of carbohydrates naturally.

## Dairy products

Milk, yoghurts (especially the low-fat and fat-free thick ones which have starchy fillers), cheese spread, dried milk ( non-fat dry milk). Note that soft cheeses have more carbohydrates in the lower-fat versions.

## Sauces, dressings and condiments

Many have sugar and or starch added, so read the labels of everything from tomato ketchup (catsup) to commercial salad cream or even bought French dressing! Blended spices, too often have starchy fillers in them and even baking powder can have some! Fresh garlic and garlic purée contain carbohydrates and so does balsamic vinegar (but most other ones have none). Watch out, too, for mustards, soy sauce, coffee whitener and even stock cubes.

## Drinks

Coffee and cocoa contain some carbohydrates. Beers, sweet wines and liqueurs have lots. Watch out for diet drinks. Unless they have 0 calories, they will probably contain some carbohydrates. Always check the labels.

# Portion Sizes – the All-important Factor

I have calculated the foods using average portions to make the book more user-friendly. To be sure of success with your diet you must stick to these portion sizes.

Until you get used to the diet and the measurements you are using, here are the exact portion sizes I am referring to in the carbohydrates counter. Remember, it's up to you not to cheat. If you give yourself larger quantities of the foods you are not supposed to be eating, you will suffer the consequences! I stress that for spoon sizes of average servings, I have used a large serving spoon, not a measuring spoon. For liquids, I have used standard measures: 1 teaspoon = 5 ml, 1 tablespoon = 15 ml.

## Prepared dishes

Whether home-made or bought ready prepared, they will have a serving size on them. For example, if a bought lasagne or a recipe cooked at home says it serves four people, '1 average serving' (as stated in the carb counter) is a quarter of the lasagne. Likewise, if it says it serves two people, '1 average serving' will be half of the dish.

Please note that brands do vary and manufacturers do change their recipes from time to time. I have taken average counts from average recipes, using both UK and American data, but I recommend you always read labels for the latest and most precise information.

| Food | Portion size given | Equivalent weight or size |
|---|---|---|
| Butter or other spreads | 1 small knob | 10 g/¼ oz/2 tsp |
| Cakes and pies | 1 average slice | ⅛ standard pie or cake<br>⅙ large pizza or quiche |
| Cereals: these vary according to type (flakes, porridge etc.) and are based on manufacturer's recommended serving size, so you can double-check on the packet. For the spoon measure, use a large serving spoon not a measuring spoon. | 3 heaped tablespoons | 50 g/2 oz or 40 g/1½ oz (muesli, heavy grains and bite-sized cereals) |
|  | 5 heaped tablespoons | 40 g/1½ oz or 30 g/1¼ oz (flakes, instant oat and puffed cereals) |
| Cheese | 1 small wedge/1 good spoonful/1 small chunk | 25 g/1 oz |
| Chocolate | 1 standard bar | One up from fun-size; the standard bars vary but are, on average, around 40 g/1½ oz |
| Croûtons | 1 heaped tablespoon | 15 g/½ oz |

| Food | Portion size given | Equivalent weight or size |
|------|-------------------|---------------------------|
| Drinks | 1 single measure | 25 ml/1 fl oz/1½ tbsp |
| | 1 double measure | 50 ml/2 fl oz/3 tbsp |
| | 1 small glass | 100 ml/3½ fl oz/scant ½ cup |
| | 1 wine glass | 120 ml/4 fl oz/½ cup |
| | 1 tumbler | 200 ml/7 fl oz/scant 1 cu |
| | 1 mug | 250 ml/8 fl oz/1 cup |
| | 1 small (beer/cider) | 300 ml/½ pt/1¼ cups |
| Fish | 1 average (piece of) fillet or steak | 175 g/6 oz |
| Fruit and vegetables (see also potatoes) | a good handful | about 25 g/1 oz |
| | 2 good tablespoons | 50 g/2 oz |
| | 3 heaped tablespoons | 100 g/4 oz |
| Ice cream | 1 scoop | 50 g/2 oz |
| Meat and poultry, roast | 2 thick slices/ 2–3 medium slices/ 4 thin slices | 100 g/4 oz |
| Meat, deli | 1 medium slice/ 1 thin slice | As purchased pre-packed |
| Noodles, all types | 1 average serving | 50 g/2 oz uncooked |
| Nuts and dried fruit | 1 small handful | 15 g/½ oz |
| Pancetta, diced | 2 level tablespoons | 50 g/2 oz |
| Pasta, all types | 1 average serving | 75 g/3 oz uncooked |

| Food | Portion size given | Equivalent weight or size |
|------|--------------------|---------------------------|
| Potatoes: | | |
| baked, skins only | 1 medium potato | 50 g/2 oz |
| boiled, roast, steamed | 2 medium pieces/ 3 small new | 100 g/4 oz |
| baked, whole | 1 large potato | 225 g/8 oz |
| Rice, all types | 1 average serving | 50 g/2 oz/¼ cup uncooked |
| Sauces and sundries | 1 level teaspoon 1 level tablespoon | 5 ml 15 ml |
| Soup | 2 ladlefuls | 200 ml/7 fl oz/scant 1 cup |
| Snacks | 1 small bag | Crisps (potato chips): 25 g/1 oz Corn snacks, chocolate peanuts etc.: 50 g/2 oz |
| Steaks | 1 medium 1 large (T-bone) | 175 g/6 oz 350 g/12 oz |

# A–Z of Carbohydrate Values

The easy-to-follow page headings and clear presentation mean that you will quickly and easily find the items you are looking for. **The shaded boxes indicate those foods you are allowed to eat on the quick-weight-loss phase of the diet.** Do remember, though, that some – particularly the vegetables – do contain carbohydrates, so you'll need to make sure you check the amounts as even small quantities will add up to more than your allowance if you are not careful.

You can make your own notes on favourite brands, recipe ideas and healthy food combinations at the end of each section.

| Food | Carbo-hydrate g | Portion size | Fat g | Protein g | Fibre | kCalories per portion |
|---|---|---|---|---|---|---|
| **Abbey crunch** biscuits (cookies) | 7 | 1 biscuit | 2 | 1 | low | 46 |
| **Absinthe** | trace | 1 single measure | trace | trace | 0 | 55 |
| **Ace** chocolate bar | 16 | 1 standard bar | 6 | 1 | low | 126 |
| **Aduki beans**, dried, soaked and boiled | 22 | 3 heaped tbsp | trace | 9 | high | 123 |
| **Advocaat** | 7 | 1 single measure | 2 | 1 | 0 | 68 |
| **Aero** chocolate bar, mint | 28 | 1 standard bar | 13 | 3 | 0 | 254 |
| Aero chocolate bar, orange | 28 | 1 standard bar | 13 | 3 | 0 | 254 |
| Aero chocolate bar, milk | 26 | 1 standard bar | 13 | 3 | 0 | 251 |
| **Afelia** (greek pork stew) | 12 | 1 average serving | 28 | 24 | low | 369 |
| **After eight mints** | 6 | 1 mint | 1 | trace | 0 | 32 |
| **Aioli** | trace | 2 level tbsp | 23 | trace | 0 | 237 |
| **Alfalfa sprouts** | 1 | 1 good handful | trace | trace | high | 7 |
| **All-bran**, dry | 11 | 25 g/1 oz/½ cup | 1 | 3 | high | 68 |
| All-bran, with semi-skimmed milk | 16 | 5 heaped tbsp | 3 | 8 | high | 139 |
| All-bran, with skimmed milk | 16 | 5 heaped tbsp | 1 | 8 | high | 123 |
| **Almond biscuits** (cookies) | 6 | 1 biscuit | 2 | 1 | low | 46 |
| **Almond danish** pastry | 46 | 1 pastry | 24 | 6 | med | 420 |
| **Almond macaroon** | 13 | 1 macaroon | 7 | 3 | med | 120 |
| **Almond paste** | 17 | 25 g/1 oz | 4 | 1 | med | 101 |
| **Almond slice** | 21 | 1 slice | 5 | 2 | low | 132 |

| Food | Carbo-hydrate g | Portion size | Fat g | Protein g | Fibre | kCalories per portion |
|------|-----------------|--------------|-------|-----------|-------|------------------------|
| **Almonds**, fresh, shelled | **2** | 25 g/1 oz/¼ cup | 14 | 5 | high | 153 |
| Almonds, ground | **trace** | 1 level tbsp | 4 | 3 | high | 46 |
| Almonds, roasted | **1** | 1 small handful | 9 | 3 | high | 95 |
| Almonds, sugared | **3** | 1 sweet (candy) | trace | trace | high | 15 |
| **Alpen**, dry | **16** | 25 g/1 oz/¼ cup | 2 | 2 | high | 91 |
| Alpen, with semi-skimmed milk | **33** | 3 heaped tbsp | 5 | 8 | high | 203 |
| Alpen, with skimmed milk | **33** | 3 heaped tbsp | 3 | 8 | high | 189 |
| Alpen, no added sugar, dry | **15** | 25 g/1 oz/¼ cup | 2 | 3 | high | 89 |
| Alpen, no added sugar, with semi-skimmed milk | **31** | 3 heaped tbsp | 5 | 9 | high | 200 |
| Alpen, no added sugar, with skimmed milk | **31** | 3 heaped tbsp | 3 | 9 | high | 184 |
| Alpen nutty crunch, dry | **16** | 25 g/1 oz/¼ cup | 2 | 2 | high | 95 |
| Alpen nutty crunch, with semi-skimmed milk | **32** | 3 heaped tbsp | 6 | 8 | high | 209 |
| Alpen nutty crunch, with skimmed milk | **32** | 3 heaped tbsp | 4 | 8 | high | 193 |
| **Alphabetti spaghetti**, canned | **28** | 1 small can | 1 | 4 | med | 135 |
| Alphabetti spaghetti, on toast | **46** | 1 small can plus 1 slice of buttered toast | 9 | 7 | med | 304 |

| Food | Carbo-hydrate g | Portion size | Fat g | Protein g | Fibre | kCalories per portion |
|---|---|---|---|---|---|---|
| **Amaretti biscuits** (cookies) | 4 | 1 biscuit | trace | trace | low | 21 |
| **Amaretto liqueur** | 7 | 1 single measure | 0 | 0 | 0 | 80 |
| **American hard gums** | 40 | 1 small tube | 0 | 2 | 0 | 135 |
| **American muffin,** plain | 24 | 1 muffin | 6 | 5 | med | 169 |
| **American pancake** | 8 | 1 pancake | 2 | 2 | low | 60 |
| **Anchovies**, canned | 0 | 1 fillet | 1 | 1 | 0 | 12 |
| Anchovies, fresh, grilled (broiled) | 0 | 1 fish | 4 | 15 | 0 | 98 |
| **Anchovy essence** (extract) | 0 | 1 level tsp | trace | 1 | 0 | 7 |
| **Anchovy paste** | trace | 1 level tbsp | 1 | 3 | 0 | 20 |
| **Angel cake** | 12 | 1 slice | trace | 1 | low | 77 |
| **Angel delight**, all flavours, made with semi-skimmed milk | 16 | 1 average serving | 4 | 3 | 0 | 115 (average) |
| Angel delight, all flavours, made with skimmed milk | 16 | 1 average serving | 2 | 3 | 0 | 105 (average) |
| Angel delight, sugar-free, all flavours, made with semi-skimmed milk | 13 | 1 average serving | 5 | 3 | 0 | 115 (average) |
| Angel delight, sugar-free, all flavours, made with skimmed milk | 13 | 1 average serving | 4 | 3 | 0 | 105 (average) |
| **Angel hair** (pasta strands), dried, boiled | 51 | 1 average serving | 2 | 8 | med | 239 |

| Food | Carbo-hydrate g | Portion size | Fat g | Protein g | Fibre | kCalories per portion |
|---|---|---|---|---|---|---|
| Angel hair, fresh, boiled | 57 | 1 average serving | 2 | 11 | med | 301 |
| **Angels on horseback** | trace | 1 oyster plus ½ rasher (slice) of bacon | 3 | 4 | 0 | 37 |
| **Anis** | trace | 1 single measure | 0 | trace | 0 | 55 |
| **Aniseed balls** | 87 | 1 small tube | trace | trace | 0 | 81 |
| **Antipasti**, mixed | 11 | 1 average serving | 13 | 24 | high | 244 |
| **Anzac biscuits** (cookies) | 4 | 1 biscuit | 5 | 2 | low | 98 |
| **Apple** | 12 | 1 med fruit | trace | trace | high | 47 |
| Apple, cooking (tart) | 9 | 1 large fruit, peeled | trace | trace | med | 35 |
| Apple, cooking, baked, sweetened | 12 | 1 large fruit | trace | 1 | high | 140 |
| Apple, dried rings | 3 | 1 ring | trace | trace | high | 13 |
| Apple, dried rings, stewed | 13 | 3 heaped tbsp | trace | trace | high | 66 |
| Apple, dried rings, stewed with sugar | 17 | 3 heaped tbsp | trace | trace | high | 106 |
| Apple, stewed | 8 | 3 heaped tbsp | trace | trace | med | 33 |
| Apple, stewed with sugar | 19 | 3 heaped tbsp | trace | trace | med | 74 |
| Apple, toffee | 66 | 1 med fruit | trace | 4 | high | 251 |
| **Apple amber** | 14 | 1 average serving | 2 | 2 | med | 340 |
| **Apple and black-currant juice drink** | 16 | 1 tumbler | trace | trace | 0 | 74 |
| **Apple and mango juice drink** | 13 | 1 tumbler | trace | 0 | 0 | 67 |

| Food | Carbo-hydrate g | Portion size | Fat g | Protein g | Fibre | kCalories per portion |
|---|---|---|---|---|---|---|
| **Apple betty** | 39 | 1 average serving | 10 | 2 | med | 260 |
| **Apple cake** | 32 | 1 average slice | 10 | 3 | med | 252 |
| **Apple charlotte** | 41 | 1 average serving | 9 | 3 | med | 263 |
| **Apple chutney** | 3 | 1 tbsp | trace | trace | low | 30 |
| **Apple croissant** | 21 | 1 croissant | 5 | 4 | med | 144 |
| **Apple crumble** | 51 | 1 average serving | 10 | 3 | med | 297 |
| **Apple danish pastry** | 51 | 1 pastry | 18 | 6 | med | 298 |
| **Apple drink,** sparkling | 19 | 1 tumbler | trace | trace | 0 | 78 |
| Apple drink, sparkling, low-cal | 2 | 1 tumbler | trace | trace | 0 | 9 |
| **Apple dumpling** | 54 | 1 dumpling | 8 | 3 | high | 287 |
| **Apple fritter** | 26 | 1 fritter | 5 | 2 | med | 136 |
| **Apple jelly** (clear conserve) | 17 | 1 level tbsp | 0 | 0 | low | 67 |
| **Apple juice** | 10 | 1 tumbler | trace | trace | low | 76 |
| Apple juice drink, diluted | 21 | 1 tumbler | trace | trace | 0 | 88 |
| **Apple pie** | 39 | 1 average slice | 14 | 3 | med | 290 |
| **Apple sauce** | 2 | 1 level tbsp | trace | trace | med | 25 |
| **Apple snow** | 19 | 1 average serving | 1 | 4 | med | 97 |
| **Apple strudel** | 29 | 1 average slice | 8 | 2 | med | 194 |
| **Apple tango** | 19 | 1 tumbler | trace | trace | 0 | 78 |
| Apple tango, light | 2 | 1 tumbler | trace | trace | 0 | 9 |
| **Apple turnover** | 31 | 1 turnover | 16 | 4 | med | 284 |
| **Apricot** | 4 | 1 fruit | trace | trace | med | 17 |

| Food | Carbo-hydrate g | Portion size | Fat g | Protein g | Fibre | kCalories per portion |
|---|---|---|---|---|---|---|
| **Apricot & almond danish pastry** | 38 | 1 pastry | 12 | 6 | med | 270 |
| **Apricot bites**, dry | 13 | 25 g/1 oz/½ cup | 1 | 3 | high | 70 |
| **Apricot bites**, with semi-skimmed milk | 27 | 3 heaped tbsp | 2 | 9 | high | 169 |
| Apricot bites, with skimmed milk | 27 | 3 heaped tbsp | 3 | 9 | high | 153 |
| **Apricot brandy** | 7 | 1 single measure | 0 | trace | 0 | 56 |
| **Apricot jam** (conserve) | 10 | 1 level tbsp | 0 | trace | 0 | 39 |
| **Apricot juice** | 20 | 1 tumbler | trace | 1 | 0 | 78 |
| **Apricot nectar** | 32 | 1 tumbler | trace | 1 | 0 | 112 |
| **Apricot sorbet** | 19 | 1 scoop | trace | trace | low | 57 |
| **Apricots**, canned in natural juice | 8 | 3 heaped tbsp | trace | trace | med | 34 |
| Apricots, canned in syrup | 16 | 3 heaped tbsp | trace | trace | med | 63 |
| Apricots, dried | 3 | 1 fruit | trace | trace | high | 15 |
| Apricots, dried, stewed | 22 | 3 heaped tbsp | trace | 1 | high | 85 |
| Apricots, dried, stewed with sugar | 29 | 3 heaped tbsp | trace | 1 | high | 113 |
| Apricots, stewed | 7 | 3 heaped tbsp | trace | 1 | med | 31 |
| Apricots, stewed with sugar | 15 | 3 heaped tbsp | trace | 1 | med | 61 |
| **Arbroath smokies**, grilled (broiled), with butter | 0 | 1 med fish | 10 | 37 | 0 | 239 |
| **Archers peach liqueur** | 8 | 1 single measure | 0 | trace | 0 | 65 |

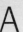

| Food | Carbo-hydrate g | Portion size | Fat g | Protein g | Fibre | kCalories per portion |
|---|---|---|---|---|---|---|
| **Arctic roll** | 16 | 1 average slice | 3 | 2 | low | 100 |
| **Arrowroot biscuits** (cookies), thin | 7 | 1 biscuit | 2 | 1 | low | 35 |
| **Artichoke**, globe, boiled | 3 | 1 med artichoke | 0 | 0 | med | 70 |
| Artichoke, with melted butter | 3 | 1 med artichoke | 13 | 1 | med | 181 |
| Artichoke hearts, canned, drained | 1 | 1 heart | trace | 1 | med | 8 |
| Artichoke vinaigrette | 3 | 1 med artichoke | 22 | 1 | med | 211 |
| Artichokes, Jerusalem, boiled | 11 | 3 heaped tbsp | 0 | 2 | high | 41 |
| **Asparagus**, canned, drained | 1 | ½ med can | trace | 3 | med | 24 |
| Asparagus, roasted in olive oil | 1 | 6 thick or 10 thin spears | 16 | 3 | med | 161 |
| Asparagus, steamed or boiled | 2 | 6 thick or 10 thin spears | 2 | 3 | med | 26 |
| Asparagus, with melted butter | 1 | 6 thick or 10 thin spears | 13 | 3 | med | 137 |
| **Asparagus quiche** | 18 | 1 average slice | 22 | 13 | med | 320 |
| **Asparagus soup**, cream of, canned | 10 | 2 ladlefuls | 10 | 2 | low | 132 |
| Asparagus soup, cream of, instant | 20 | 1 mug | 6 | 1 | low | 143 |
| Asparagus soup, home-made | 7 | 2 ladlefuls | 14 | 3 | high | 167 |

| Food | Carbo-hydrate g | Portion size | Fat g | Protein g | Fibre | kCalories per portion |
|------|------|------|------|------|------|------|
| **Aubergine** (egg-plant), fried (sautéed) in oil | 3 | ¼ med aubergine | 32 | 1 | med | 302 |
| Aubergine, steamed or boiled | 3 | ¼ med aubergine | trace | 1 | med | 28 |
| Aubergine, stuffed with meat | **28** | ½ med aubergine | 24 | 46 | med | 510 |
| Aubergine, stuffed with savoury rice | **26** | ½ med aubergine | 14 | 8 | high | 523 |
| **Aubergine dip** | 4 | 2 tbsp | 1 | 1 | med | 20 |
| **Austrian coffee cake** | 41 | 1 average slice | 32 | 5 | low | 488 |
| **Austrian smoked cheese** | trace | 25 g/1 oz | 3 | 4 | 0 | 60 |
| **Avgolemono soup** | 5 | 2 ladlefuls | 2 | 3 | low | 74 |
| **Avocado** | 3 | 1 med fruit | 29 | 3 | med | 286 |
| Avocado, baked, with tomato and cheese | 4 | ½ med avocado | 18 | 5 | med | 196 |
| Avocado, with prawns (shrimp) in cocktail sauce | 2 | ½ med avocado | 32 | 13 | med | 356 |
| **Avocado vinaigrette** | 1 | ½ med avocado | 25 | 1 | med | 240 |

| Food | Carbo-hydrate g | Portion size | Fat g | Protein g | Fibre | kCalories per portion |
|---|---|---|---|---|---|---|
| **Babybel cheese** | 0 | 1 cheese | 4 | 4 | 0 | 53 |
| **Bacardi** | trace | 1 single measure | trace | trace | 0 | 50 |
| Bacardi and coke | 6 | 1 single measure plus 1 mixer | 0 | trace | 0 | 94 |
| Bacardi and diet coke | trace | 1 single measure plus 1 mixer | 0 | trace | 0 | 56 |
| **Baclava** | 40 | 1 pastry | 17 | 5 | med | 322 |
| **Bacon**, back, lean, fried (sautéed) | 0 | 1 rasher (slice) | 16 | 13 | 0 | 133 |
| Bacon, back, lean, grilled (broiled) | 0 | 1 rasher | 8 | 12 | 0 | 117 |
| Bacon, joint, boiled | 0 | 2 med slices | 27 | 20 | 0 | 325 |
| Bacon, joint, honey-roasted | 4 | 2 med slices | 27 | 20 | 0 | 346 |
| Bacon, streaky, fried | 0 | 1 rasher | 13 | 7 | 0 | 149 |
| Bacon, streaky, grilled | 0 | 1 rasher | 11 | 7 | 0 | 127 |
| **Bacon and egg quiche** | 17 | 1 average slice | 31 | 15 | low | 387 |
| **Bacon and egg mcmuffin** | 26 | 1 muffin | 18 | 20 | med | 346 |
| **Bacon and mushroom pizza**, deep-pan | 35 | 1 large slice | 16 | 10 | med | 340 |
| Bacon and mushroom pizza, thin-crust | 25 | 1 large slice | 15 | 10 | med | 290 |
| **Bacon cheeseburger** | 27 | 1 burger | 22 | 24 | low | 400 |
| **Bacon sandwiches** | 34 | 1 round | 32 | 30 | med | 538 |

| Food | Carbo-hydrate g | Portion size | Fat g | Protein g | Fibre | kCalories per portion |
|---|---|---|---|---|---|---|
| **Bagel** | 44 | 1 bagel | 3 | 7 | med | 228 |
| **Bagna cauda** | 0 | 1 individual pot | 52 | 6 | 0 | 499 |
| **Baguette** | 75 | 1 small | 2 | 11 | med | 364 |
| **Bailey's irish cream** | 6 | 1 single measure | 4 | trace | 0 | 80 |
| **Baked alaska** | 62 | 1 average serving | 8 | 8 | low | 339 |
| **Baked beans** | 31 | 1 small can | 1 | 10 | high | 168 |
| Baked beans, barbecued | 30 | 1 small can | 1 | 10 | high | 164 |
| Baked beans, on toast | 49 | 1 small can plus 1 slice of toast | 10 | 14 | high | 323 |
| Baked beans, reduced-sugar and reduced-salt | 25 | 1 small can | 1 | 11 | high | 146 |
| Baked beans, reduced-sugar and reduced-salt, on toast | 43 | 1 small can plus 1 slice of toast | 10 | 14 | high | 301 |
| Baked beans, with bacon | 26 | 1 small can plus 2 rashers (slices) of bacon | 3 | 12 | high | 182 |
| Baked beans, with burgers, canned | 26 | 1 small can | 6 | 13 | high | 206 |
| Baked beans, with sausages, canned | 26 | 1 small can | 9 | 10 | high | 220 |
| Baked beans, with vegetarian sausages, canned | 63 | 1 small can | trace | 11 | high | 240 |
| **Bakewell slice** | 22 | 1 average slice | 7 | 1 | med | 156 |
| **Bakewell tart** | 37 | 1 average slice | 15 | 4 | med | 297 |
| **Balsamic vinegar** | 1 | 1 tsp | 0 | trace | 0 | 1 |

| Food | Carbo-hydrate g | Portion size | Fat g | Protein g | Fibre | kCalories per portion |
|------|-----------------|--------------|-------|-----------|-------|------------------------|
| **Bamboo shoots** | trace | 2 good tbsp | trace | 1 | med | 6 |
| **Banana** | 23 | 1 med fruit | trace | 1 | med | 95 |
| Banana, dried slices | 9 | 1 small handful | 5 | trace | med | 78 |
| **Banana bread** | 45 | 1 average slice | 7 | 2 | med | 246 |
| **Banana custard** | 8 | 5 tbsp | 1 | 1 | 0 | 50 |
| **Banana flambé** | 28 | 1 med banana | 8 | 1 | med | 250 |
| **Banana fritter** | 33 | 1 fritter | 5 | 3 | med | 175 |
| **Banana milkshake**, fresh, made with semi-skimmed milk | 31 | 1 tumbler | 3 | 6 | med | 163 |
| Banana milkshake, fresh, made with skimmed milk | 31 | 1 tumbler | trace | 6 | med | 144 |
| **Banana sandwiches** | 57 | 1 round | 17 | 7 | med | 399 |
| **Banana split** | 77 | 1 average serving | 16 | 10 | med | 481 |
| **Bananabix**, dry | 18 | 25 g/1 oz/½ cup | trace | 2 | high | 92 |
| Bananabix, with semi-skimmed milk | 35 | 3 heaped tbsp | 4 | 8 | high | 207 |
| Bananabix, with skimmed milk | 35 | 3 heaped tbsp | 3 | 8 | high | 191 |
| **Bangers and mash** | 43 | 2 sausages , 4 heaped tbspfuls mash | 20 | 17 | med | 462 |
| **Banoffee pie** | 68 | 1 average slice | 23 | 10 | med | 574 |
| **Barbecue sauce** | 1 | 1 level tbsp | trace | trace | 0 | 11 |
| **Barbecued baked beans** | 30 | 1 small can | 1 | 10 | high | 164 |
| **Barbecued chicken** | 1 | 1 chicken portion | 10 | 46 | 0 | 287 |

| Food | Carbo-hydrate g | Portion size | Fat g | Protein g | Fibre | kCalories per portion |
|---|---|---|---|---|---|---|
| **Barbecued pork chop** | 1 | 1 chop | 9 | 28 | 0 | 210 |
| **Barbecued spare ribs** | 2 | 2 ribs | 16 | 25 | 0 | 288 |
| **Barley sugar** | 24 | 1 stick | 0 | trace | 0 | 96 |
| **Barley water,** all flavours | 9 | 1 tumbler | trace | trace | 0 | 40 (average) |
| **Barley water,** all flavours, no added sugar | 1 | 1 tumbler | trace | trace | 0 | 6 (average) |
| **Barley wine** | 11 | 1 small bottle | trace | 1 | 0 | 120 |
| **Bass,** fried (sautéed), in seasoned flour | 5 | 1 piece of fillet | 12 | 32 | low | 261 |
| **Bass,** grilled (broiled) | 0 | 1 piece of fillet | 2 | 31 | 0 | 142 |
| **Bass,** poached | 0 | 1 piece of fillet | 2 | 32 | 0 | 141 |
| Bass, stuffed, baked | 1 | 1 serving | 4 | 32 | low | 182 |
| **Bath bun** | 45 | 1 bun | 15 | 8 | med | 263 |
| **Bath olivers** | 8 | 1 biscuit (cookie) | 2 | 1 | low | 50 |
| **Battenburg cake** | 50 | 1 average slice | 17 | 6 | med | 370 |
| **Bavarian smoked cheese** | trace | 25 g/1 oz | 3 | 4 | 0 | 60 |
| **Bavarois,** all flavours | 17 | 1 average serving | 23 | 7 | 0 | 308 (average) |
| **Bean and cheese enchiladas** | 82 | 2 enchiladas | 14 | 28 | high | 547 |
| **Bean salad** | 12 | 3 heaped tbsp | 5 | 4 | high | 120 |
| **Beanburger,** spicy | 4 | 1 burger | 6 | 9 | med | 112 |
| **Beans** *See individual varieties,* e.g. Runner beans | | | | | | |

| Food | Carbo-hydrate g | Portion size | Fat g | Protein g | Fibre | kCalories per portion |
|---|---|---|---|---|---|---|
| **Beansprouts** | 1 | 1 good handful | trace | 1 | high | 8 |
| **Béarnaise sauce** | 7 | 5 level tbsp | 27 | 3 | low | 275 |
| **Béchamel sauce,** made with semi-skimmed milk | 8 | 5 level tbsp | 6 | 3 | low | 96 |
| Beef, boiled | 0 | 2 thick slices | 24 | 28 | 0 | 326 |
| Beef, corned | 0 | 1 thin slice | 3 | 7 | 0 | 54 |
| Beef, grillsteak, grilled (broiled) | 8 | 1 steak | 12 | 11 | low | 185 |
| Beef, minced (ground), in gravy, canned | 14 | ½ large can | 11 | 19 | 0 | 230 |
| Beef, minced, lean, stewed | 0 | 1 average serving | 15 | 23 | 0 | 229 |
| Beef, roast, lean | 0 | 4 thin slices | 19 | 28 | 0 | 225 |
| Beef, steak See Steak | | | | | | |
| Beef, stewed in gravy | 0 | 1 average serving | 16 | 47 | 0 | 335 |
| Beef, stewed in gravy, canned | 8 | ½ large can | 10 | 32 | 0 | 254 |
| **Beef and cheese enchiladas** | 60 | 2 enchiladas | 36 | 24 | low | 644 |
| **Beef and tomato soup,** canned | 10 | 2 ladlefuls | 2 | 5 | low | 88 |
| Beef and tomato soup, instant | 15 | 1 mug | 1 | 1 | 0 | 72 |
| **Beef and vegetable stir-fry** | 71 | 1 average serving | 5 | 26 | high | 433 |
| **Beef broth,** canned | 13 | 2 ladlefuls | 1 | 4 | med | 76 |

| Food | Carbo-hydrate g | Portion size | Fat g | Protein g | Fibre | kCalories per portion |
|---|---|---|---|---|---|---|
| **Beef carbonnade** (in beer) | 15 | 1 average serving | 21 | 30 | low | 384 |
| **Beef casserole** | 13 | 1 average serving | 21 | 28 | med | 360 |
| **Beef chop suey** | 34 | 1 average serving | 6 | 23 | med | 297 |
| **Beef chow mein** | 43 | 1 average serving | 18 | 19 | high | 408 |
| **Beef consommé,** canned | 1 | 2 ladlefuls | trace | 3 | 0 | 14 |
| Beef consommé, jellied | 1 | 2 ladlefuls | trace | 4 | 0 | 21 |
| **Beef curry,** home-made | 10 | 1 average serving | 77 | 37 | med | 905 |
| Beef curry, home-made, with rice | 66 | 1 average serving | 79 | 42 | med | 1153 |
| Beef curry, retail | 19 | 1 average serving | 18 | 40 | med | 411 |
| Beef curry, retail, with rice | 82 | 1 average serving | 19 | 43 | med | 657 |
| **Beef fajitas** | 79 | 2 fajitas | 8 | 40 | med | 528 |
| **Beef goulash** | 16 | 1 average serving | 22 | 28 | med | 406 |
| **Beef in** oyster sauce | 10 | 1 average serving | 8 | 24 | low | 204 |
| **Beef kheema** | 1 | 1 average serving | 75 | 36 | low | 826 |
| **Beef koftas** | 4 | 1 average serving | 35 | 28 | low | 441 |
| **Beef olives** | 20 | 2 olives | 18 | 58 | low | 494 |
| **Beef pie** | 32 | 1 individual pie | 28 | 18 | low | 460 |
| **Beef pot roast,** with vegetables | 14 | 1 average serving | 15 | 44 | med | 420 |
| **Beef risotto** | 54 | 1 average serving | 29 | 16 | low | 452 |
| **Beef satay** | 6 | 1 skewer | 11 | 25 | low | 222 |

| Food | Carbo-hydrate g | Portion size | Fat g | Protein g | Fibre | kCalories per portion |
|---|---|---|---|---|---|---|
| **Beef sausages,** thick, fried (sautéed) | 6 | 1 sausage | 7 | 5 | low | **108** |
| Beef sausages, thick, grilled (broiled) | 6 | 1 sausage | 7 | 5 | low | 106 |
| Beef sausages, thin, fried | 4 | 1 sausage | 4 | 3 | low | 54 |
| Beef sausages, thin, grilled | 4 | 1 sausage | 4 | 3 | low | 53 |
| **Beef spread** | 2 | 1 level tbsp | 3 | 1 | low | 35 |
| **Beef steak pudding** | 57 | 1 average serving | 37 | 33 | med | 684 |
| **Beef stew** | 13 | 1 average serving | 21 | 28 | med | 360 |
| **Beef stroganoff** | 8 | 1 average serving | 25 | 22 | med | 361 |
| **Beef teriyaki** | 2 | 1 average serving | 4 | 18 | low | 128 |
| **Beef wellington** | 23 | 1 average serving | 33 | 37 | low | 527 |
| **Beef with mushrooms,** Chinese | 44 | 1 average serving | 6 | 37 | low | 320 |
| **Beef with pineapple**, Chinese | 47 | 1 average serving | 6 | 23 | low | 337 |
| *See also* Boeuf | | | | | | |
| **Beefburger,** fried (sautéed) | trace | 1 burger | 11 | 6 | 0 | 125 |
| Beefburger, grilled (broiled) | trace | 1 burger | 11 | 6 | 0 | 122 |
| Beefburger, in a bun, quarterpounder | 27 | 1 burger in a bun | 15 | 22 | med | 321 |
| Beefburger, in a bun, small | 23 | 1 burger in a bun | 13 | 11 | med | 246 |
| **Beer**, bitter | 7 | 1 small | trace | 1 | 0 | 96 |

| Food | Carbo-hydrate g | Portion size | Fat g | Protein g | Fibre | kCalories per portion |
|---|---|---|---|---|---|---|
| Beer, extra-strength | 18 | 1 small | trace | 2 | 0 | 216 |
| Beer, pale ale | 6 | 1 small | trace | 1 | 0 | 96 |
| Beerwurst | trace | 1 med slice | 4 | 3 | 0 | 55 |
| Beetroot (red beet) | 7 | 1 med | trace | 2 | med | 36 |
| Beetroot, boiled | 9 | 1 med | trace | 2 | med | 46 |
| Beetroot, pickled | 6 | 5 slices | trace | 1 | med | 28 |
| Bel paese cheese | trace | 1 small wedge | 7 | 5 | 0 | 87 |
| Belgian bun | 30 | 1 bun | 5 | 5 | low | 192 |
| Belgian endive *See* Chicory | | | | | | |
| Belgian ham, dry-cured | 0 | 1 thin slice | 1 | 4 | 0 | 21 |
| Bell pepper *See* Pepper | | | | | | |
| Benedictine | 6 | 1 single measure | 0 | 0 | 0 | 90 |
| Big bar ace | 25 | 1 standard bar | 10 | 2 | low | 204 |
| Big breakfast | 40 | 1 meal | 36 | 26 | high | 591 |
| Big fish sandwich | 59 | 1 bun | 43 | 23 | high | 720 |
| Big mac | 44 | 1 burger | 23 | 27 | high | 493 |
| Bigarde sauce | 10 | 5 level tbsp | 4 | 5 | low | 123 |
| Biscotti | 6 | 1 biscuit (cookie) | 1 | 1 | low | 39 |
| Biscuits (cookies), chocolate, full-coated | 17 | 1 biscuit | 7 | 1 | low | 131 |
| Biscuits, chocolate, half-coated | 11 | 1 biscuit | 4 | 1 | low | 84 |
| Biscuits, cream-filled | 10 | 1 biscuit | 4 | 1 | low | 77 |
| Biscuits, semi-sweet | 7 | 1 biscuit | 2 | 1 | low | 46 |

| Food | Carbo-hydrate g | Portion size | Fat g | Protein g | Fibre | kCalories per portion |
|------|-----------------|--------------|-------|-----------|-------|----------------------|
| Biscuits, short, sweet | 6 | 1 biscuit | 2 | 1 | low | 47 |
| Biscuits, wafer, cream-filled | 5 | 1 biscuit | 3 | trace | low | 39 |
| *See also individual names, e.g.* Hobnob | | | | | | |
| **Bitter lemon**, sparkling | 16 | 1 tumbler | 0 | trace | 0 | 68 |
| **Bitter orange**, sparkling | 16 | 1 tumbler | 0 | trace | 0 | 68 |
| **Black bean sauce** | 3 | 1 level tbsp | trace | 1 | 0 | 22 |
| **Black beans**, dried, soaked and cooked | 18 | 3 heaped tbsp | trace | trace | high | **103** |
| **Black cherries**, canned in syrup | 18 | 3 heaped tbsp | trace | 0 | low | 71 |
| **Black cherry cheesecake** | 33 | 1 average slice | 11 | 6 | low | 242 |
| **Black cherry jam** (conserve) | 10 | 1 level tbsp | 0 | trace | 0 | 39 |
| Black cherry jam, reduced-sugar | 5 | 1 level tbsp | 0 | trace | 0 | 6 |
| **Black forest gateau** | 65 | 1 average slice | 18 | 7 | low | 432 |
| **Black forest ham** | trace | 1 thin slice | 2 | 4 | 0 | 29 |
| **Black gram**, boiled | 7 | 1 average serving | trace | 4 | low | 45 |
| **Black jack chew** sweets (candies) | 3 | 1 sweet | trace | 0 | 0 | 15 |
| **Black pudding**, fried (sautéed) | 15 | 2 thick slices | 22 | 13 | low | 305 |
| **Black velvet** | 5 | 1 cocktail | 0 | 1 | 0 | 168 |
| **Blackberries** | 5 | 3 heaped tbsp | trace | 1 | high | 25 |

| Food | Carbo-hydrate g | Portion size | Fat g | Protein g | Fibre | kCalories per portion |
|---|---|---|---|---|---|---|
| Blackberries, stewed | 4 | 3 heaped tbsp | trace | 1 | med | 21 |
| Blackberries, stewed with sugar | 14 | 3 heaped tbsp | trace | 1 | med | 56 |
| **Blackberry and apple crumble** | 51 | 1 average serving | 10 | 3 | med | 297 |
| **Blackberry and apple pie** | 11 | 1 average slice | 39 | 3 | med | 281 |
| **Blackberry jam** (conserve) | 10 | 1 level tbsp | 0 | trace | 0 | 39 |
| **Blackcurrant and apple pie** | 56 | 1 average slice | 16 | 3 | med | 378 |
| **Blackcurrant and apple squash,** diluted | 15 | 1 tumbler | 0 | 0 | 0 | 58 |
| **Blackcurrant cheesecake** | 38 | 1 average slice | 12 | 3 | low | 260 |
| **Blackcurrant cordial,** diluted | 27 | 1 tumbler | 0 | trace | 0 | 103 |
| **Blackcurrant crumble** | 51 | 1 average serving | 10 | 3 | med | 298 |
| **Blackcurrant jam** (conserve) | 10 | 1 level tbsp | 0 | trace | 0 | 39 |
| Blackcurrant jam, reduced-sugar | 5 | 1 level tbsp | 0 | trace | 0 | 6 |
| **Blackcurrant juice drink** | 32 | 1 tumbler | trace | trace | 0 | 120 |
| **Blackcurrant pastilles** | 32 | 1 small tube | 0 | 3 | 0 | 131 |
| **Blackcurrant pie** | 34 | 1 average slice | 13 | 3 | med | 282 |
| **Blackcurrant sorbet** | 17 | 1 scoop | trace | trace | 0 | 65 |

| Food | Carbo-hydrate g | Portion size | Fat g | Protein g | Fibre | kCalories per portion |
|---|---|---|---|---|---|---|
| **Blackcurrants** | 7 | 3 heaped tbsp | trace | 1 | high | 28 |
| Blackcurrants, canned in natural juice | 8 | 3 heaped tbsp | trace | 1 | med | 31 |
| Blackcurrants, canned in syrup | 18 | 3 heaped tbsp | trace | 1 | med | 72 |
| Blackcurrants, stewed with sugar | 15 | 3 heaped tbsp | trace | 1 | med | 58 |
| **Black-eyed beans**, dried, soaked and cooked | 20 | 3 heaped tbsp | 1 | 9 | high | 116 |
| **Blancmange** | 23 | 1 average serving | 6 | 5 | low | 165 |
| **Blewits**, fried (sautéed) | trace | 2 good tbsp | 8 | 1 | low | 78 |
| Blewits, stewed | trace | 2 good tbsp | trace | 1 | low | 6 |
| **Blinis** | 8 | 1 pancake | 2 | 2 | low | 60 |
| **Blintzes** | 11 | 1 pancake | 1 | 8 | low | 86 |
| **Bloater**, grilled (broiled) | 0 | 1 med fish | 19 | 31 | 0 | 298 |
| **Bloater paste** | 1 | 1 level tsp | trace | trace | low | 5 |
| **Bloody mary** | 3 | 1 cocktail | trace | 1 | low | 69 |
| **Bloomer loaf** | 15 | 1 med slice | 1 | 3 | low | 70 |
| **BLT** | 34 | 1 round | 35 | 30 | med | 650 |
| **Blue brie cheese** | trace | 1 small wedge | 10 | 4 | 0 | 106 |
| **Blue chartreuse** | 7 | 1 single measure | 0 | trace | 0 | 78 |
| **Blue cheese dip** | trace | 1 small pot | 12 | 1 | 0 | 145 |
| **Blue cheese dressing** | 1 | 1 level tbsp | 8 | 1 | 0 | 77 |

| Food | Carbo-hydrate g | Portion size | Fat g | Protein g | Fibre | kCalories per portion |
|---|---|---|---|---|---|---|
| Blue cheese dressing, low-calorie | 2 | 1 level tbsp | 1 | trace | 0 | 16 |
| **Blue riband** chocolate wafer | 13 | 1 standard bar | 6 | 1 | low | 108 |
| **Blue stilton cheese** | trace | 1 small wedge | 9 | 6 | 0 | 103 |
| **Blueberries** | 14 | 3 heaped tbsp | trace | 1 | med | 56 |
| Blueberries, canned in syrup | 22 | 3 heaped tbsp | trace | 1 | med | 88 |
| Blueberries, dried | 12 | 1 small handful | trace | trace | high | 44 |
| Blueberries, stewed | 12 | 3 heaped tbsp | trace | trace | med | 51 |
| Blueberries, stewed with sugar | 22 | 3 heaped tbsp | trace | trace | med | 81 |
| **Blueberry buster muffin** | 47 | 1 muffin | 21 | 4 | med | 408 |
| **Blueberry muffin** | 38 | 1 large muffin | 14 | 5 | med | 294 |
| **Blueberry pie** | 39 | 1 average slice | 14 | 3 | med | 290 |
| **Bluefish**, grilled (broiled) | 0 | 1 med fillet | 6 | 30 | 0 | 186 |
| **Boasters** biscuits (cookies), all flavours | 20 | 1 biscuit | 5 | 1 | low | 90 (average) |
| **Bockwurst** | trace | 1 sausage | 18 | 9 | 0 | 199 |
| **Boeuf bourguignon** | 7 | 1 average serving | 33 | 31 | low | 450 |
| **Boeuf en daube** | 14 | 1 average serving | 13 | 39 | med | 351 |
| *See also* Beef | | | | | | |
| **Boiled beef with carrots and dumplings** | 29 | 1 average serving | 26 | 36 | med | 474 |
| **Boiled sweets** (candies) | 5 | 1 sweet | trace | trace | 0 | 15 |

| Food | Carbo-hydrate g | Portion size | Fat g | Protein g | Fibre | kCalories per portion |
|---|---|---|---|---|---|---|
| Bologna sausage | trace | 1 med slice | 5 | 3 | 0 | 57 |
| Bolognese sauce | 5 | 5 level tbsp | 17 | 12 | low | 217 |
| Bolony sausage | trace | 1 med slice | 5 | 3 | 0 | 57 |
| Bombay mix snack | 2 | 1 small handful | 5 | 1 | high | 75 |
| Bon bel cheese | 0 | 1 small wedge | 6 | 6 | 0 | 78 |
| Bon-bons | 6 | 1 sweet (candy) | trace | 0 | 0 | 28 |
| Bonito, grilled (broiled) | 0 | 1 piece of fillet | 7 | 34 | 0 | 195 |
| Boost chocolate bar | 34 | 1 standard bar | 16 | 3 | low | 295 |
| Bordelaise sauce | 2 | 5 level tbsp | 4 | 5 | 0 | 133 |
| Borlotti beans, canned, drained | 8 | 3 heaped tbsp | trace | 5 | high | 112 |
| Borlotti beans, dried, soaked and cooked | 18 | 3 heaped tbsp | 1 | 6 | high | 116 |
| Bortsch | 1 | 2 ladlefuls | 1 | 3 | high | 25 |
| Bortsch, jellied | 1 | 2 ladlefuls | 1 | 9 | high | 50 |
| Boston baked beans | 26 | 1 average serving | 1 | 7 | high | 133 |
| Boudoir biscuits (lady fingers) | 6 | 1 finger | 1 | 1 | low | 40 |
| Bouillabaisse | 21 | 2 ladlefuls | 2 | 16 | med | 159 |
| Bouillabaise with rouille | 23 | 2 ladlefuls | 17 | 17 | med | 310 |
| Bounty bar, milk chocolate | 32 | 1 standard bar | 15 | 3 | low | 289 |
| Bounty bar, plain (semi-sweet) chocolate | 33 | 1 standard bar | 15 | 2 | low | 276 |
| Bounty, ice cream bar | 24 | 1 standard bar | 21 | 4 | low | 299 |

| Food | Carbo-hydrate g | Portion size | Fat g | Protein g | Fibre | kCalories per portion |
|------|------|------|------|------|------|------|
| **Bourbon** | **trace** | 1 single measure | 0 | trace | 0 | 60 |
| **Bourbon biscuits** (cookies) | **9** | 1 biscuit | 3 | 1 | low | 63 |
| **Bournville** chocolate | **30** | 1 standard bar | 13 | 2 | 0 | 250 |
| **Bournvita**, made with semi-skimmed milk | **19** | 1 mug | 4 | 9 | low | 145 |
| Bournvita, made with skimmed milk | 20 | 1 mug | 2 | 9 | low | 137 |
| **Boursin cheese**, all flavours | **1** | 1 good spoonful | 7 | 2 | 0 | 77 (average) |
| Boursin, light, all flavours | 1 | 1 good spoonful | 2 | 2 | 0 | 28 (average) |
| **Bovril** | **trace** | 1 level tsp | trace | 2 | 0 | 3 |
| **Bran**, oat | **9** | 1 level tbsp | 1 | 2 | high | 51 |
| Bran, wheat | 4 | 1 level tbsp | 1 | 2 | high | 31 |
| **Bran muffin** | **24** | 1 muffin | 6 | 4 | high | 163 |
| **Brandy** | **trace** | 1 single measure | 0 | trace | 0 | 55 |
| **Brandy alexander** | **6** | 1 cocktail | 18 | trace | 0 | 270 |
| **Brandy butter** | **8** | 1 level tbsp | 4 | trace | 0 | 73 |
| **Brandy sauce**, made with semi-skimmed milk | **5** | 5 level tbsp | 2 | 1 | low | 50 |
| Brandy sauce, made with skimmed milk | 5 | 5 level tbsp | trace | 1 | low | 47 |
| **Brandy snaps** | **10** | 1 snap | 2 | trace | low | 57 |
| **Brandy sour** | **trace** | 1 cocktail | trace | trace | 0 | 57 |
| **Branflakes**, dry | **16** | 25 g/1 oz/½ cup | 1 | 2 | high | 80 |

| Food | Carbo-hydrate g | Portion size | Fat g | Protein g | Fibre | kCalories per portion |
|---|---|---|---|---|---|---|
| Branflakes, with semi-skimmed milk | 33 | 5 heaped tbsp | 3 | 8 | high | 185 |
| Branflakes, with skimmed milk | 33 | 5 heaped tbsp | 1 | 8 | high | 169 |
| Branflakes, with sultanas (golden raisins), dry | 16 | 25 g/1 oz/½ cup | trace | 2 | high | 80 |
| Branflakes, with sultanas, with skimmed milk | 33 | 5 heaped tbsp | 1 | 8 | high | 169 |
| Branflakes, with sultanas, with semi-skimmed milk | 33 | 5 heaped tbsp | 3 | 8 | high | 185 |
| **Bratwurst**, fried (sautéed) | **2** | 1 sausage | 22 | 12 | 0 | 256 |
| **Brazil nut**, shelled | **trace** | 1 nut | 3 | 1 | high | 23 |
| **Brazil nut toffee** | **5** | 1 toffee | 2 | trace | low | 39 |
| **Brazils, chocolate** | **3** | 1 sweet (candy) | 4 | 1 | high | 49 |
| **Bread**, brown, medium-sliced | **16** | 1 slice | 1 | 3 | med | 78 |
| Bread, brown, medium-sliced, toasted | 16 | 1 slice | 1 | 3 | med | 80 |
| Bread, brown, thick-sliced | 22 | 1 slice | 1 | 4 | med | 109 |
| Bread, brown, thin-sliced | 13 | 1 slice | 1 | 2 | med | 65 |
| Bread, granary, medium-sliced | 18 | 1 slice | 1 | 4 | med | 94 |
| Bread, granary, medium-sliced, toasted | 18 | 1 slice | 1 | 4 | med | 96 |

| Food | Carbo-hydrate g | Portion size | Fat g | Protein g | Fibre | kCalories per portion |
|---|---|---|---|---|---|---|
| Bread, granary, thick-sliced | 23 | 1 slice | 2 | 5 | med | 117 |
| Bread, softgrain, medium-sliced | 15 | 1 slice | 1 | 3 | med | 76 |
| Bread, softgrain, medium-sliced, toasted | 18 | 1 slice | 1 | 3 | med | 85 |
| Bread, softgrain, thick-sliced | 21 | 1 slice | 1 | 5 | med | 106 |
| Bread, white, medium-sliced | 17 | 1 slice | trace | 3 | low | 78 |
| Bread, white, medium-sliced, toasted | 18 | 1 slice | trace | 3 | low | 81 |
| Bread, white, thick-sliced | 23 | 1 slice | trace | 4 | low | 108 |
| Bread, white, thin-sliced | 14 | 1 slice | trace | 2 | low | 65 |
| Bread, wholemeal, medium-sliced | 15 | 1 slice | 1 | 3 | high | 77 |
| Bread, wholemeal, medium-sliced, toasted | 15 | 1 slice | 1 | 3 | high | 79 |
| Bread, wholemeal, thick-sliced | 21 | 1 slice | 1 | 5 | high | 107 |
| Bread, wholemeal, thin-sliced | 12 | 1 slice | 1 | 3 | high | 64 |
| Bread, with butter | 17 | 1 med slice | 9 | 3 | low | 152 (average) |
| Bread, with low-fat spread | 17 | 1 med slice | 4 | 3 | low | 117 (average) |
| **Bread pudding** | 50 | 1 average serving | 10 | 6 | med | 297 |

| Food | Carbo-hydrate g | Portion size | Fat g | Protein g | Fibre | kCalories per portion |
|---|---|---|---|---|---|---|
| **Bread and butter pudding** | 31 | 1 average serving | 13 | 10 | low | 280 |
| **Bread roll**, baton | 38 | 1 roll | 1 | 6 | med | 182 |
| Bread roll, brown | 26 | 1 roll | 2 | 5 | med | 134 |
| Bread roll, crusty | 29 | 1 roll | 2 | 5 | low | 140 |
| Bread roll, finger | 21 | 1 roll | 2 | 4 | low | 107 |
| Bread roll, granary | 23 | 1 roll | 1 | 5 | med | 117 |
| Bread roll, hamburger bun | 24 | 1 bun | 2 | 4 | low | 132 |
| Bread roll, soft white bap | 26 | 1 roll | 2 | 5 | low | 134 |
| Bread roll, starch-reduced | 10 | 1 roll | trace | 2 | low | 50 |
| Bread roll, wholemeal | 24 | 1 roll | 1 | 4 | high | 120 |
| Bread roll, with butter | 29 | 1 roll | 9 | 13 | low | 214 (average) |
| Bread roll, with low-fat spread | 29 | 1 roll | 5 | 14 | low | 179 (average) |
| **Bread sauce**, made with semi-skimmed milk | 2 | 1 level tbsp | trace | 1 | low | 14 |
| Bread sauce, made with skimmed milk | 2 | 1 level tbsp | trace | 1 | low | 12 |
| **Breadfruit** | 104 | 1 med fruit | trace | 4 | high | 396 |
| Breadfruit, canned, drained | 16 | 3 heaped tbsp | trace | 1 | med | 66 |
| **Breadsticks** | 3 | 1 stick | trace | 1 | low | 20 |
| **Breakaway** chocolate bar, caramac | 13 | 1 standard bar | 7 | 1 | low | 125 |

| Food | Carbo-hydrate g | Portion size | Fat g | Protein g | Fibre | kCalories per portion |
|---|---|---|---|---|---|---|
| Breakaway, milk | 14 | 1 standard bar | 6 | 1 | low | 114 |
| **Breakfast compôte**, canned | 17 | 3 heaped tbsp | trace | trace | high | 73 |
| **Bream**, fried (sautéed) in seasoned flour | 5 | 1 piece of fillet | 12 | 32 | low | 261 |
| Bream, grilled (broiled) | 0 | 1 piece of fillet | 2 | 31 | 0 | 142 |
| Bream, poached | 0 | 1 piece of fillet | 2 | 32 | 0 | 141 |
| **Bresaola** | trace | 1 thin slice | trace | 3 | 0 | 15 |
| **Bresse bleu cheese** | trace | 1 small wedge | 10 | 4 | 0 | 106 |
| **Brie cheese** | trace | 1 small wedge | 7 | 5 | 0 | 80 |
| **Brill**, fried (sautéed) in egg and breadcrumbs | 13 | 1 piece of fillet | 20 | 27 | low | 342 |
| Brill, grilled (broiled) | 0 | 1 piece of fillet | 3 | 23 | 0 | 126 |
| Brill, poached | 0 | 1 piece of fillet | 2 | 25 | 0 | 125 |
| **Brioche** | 22 | 1 brioche | 4 | 4 | low | 140 |
| **Brisket of beef**, boiled | 0 | 2 thick slices | 24 | 28 | 0 | 326 |
| **Broad (fava) beans**, boiled | 6 | 3 heaped tbsp | 1 | 5 | high | 48 |
| Broad beans, canned, drained | 13 | 3 heaped tbsp | trace | 6 | high | 77 |
| Broad beans, frozen, cooked | 12 | 3 heaped tbsp | 1 | 8 | high | 81 |
| **Broccoli**, steamed or boiled | 2 | 4 med florets | 1 | 4 | med | 33 |
| **Broccoli and cauliflower soup**, instant | 8 | 1 mug | 2 | 1 | low | 59 |

| Food | Carbo-hydrate g | Portion size | Fat g | Protein g | Fibre | kCalories per portion |
|------|-----------------|--------------|-------|-----------|-------|------------------------|
| Broccoli and cauliflower soup, packet | 15 | 2 ladlefuls | 5 | 2 | med | 110 |
| **Broccoli and cheese quiche** | 18 | 1 large slice | 22 | 13 | low | 320 |
| **Broccoli and cheese soup**, canned | 9 | 2 ladlefuls | 7 | 4 | med | 132 |
| Broccoli and cheese soup, home-made | 21 | 2 ladlefuls | 6 | 9 | high | 169 |
| **Broccoli in cheese sauce**, made with semi-skimmed milk | 9 | 1 average serving | 11 | 10 | med | 167 |
| Broccoli in cheese sauce, made with skimmed milk | 9 | 1 average serving | 9 | 10 | med | 157 |
| **Broccoli soup** | 21 | 2 ladlefuls | 2 | 6 | high | 118 |
| **Brown ale** | 9 | 1 small | trace | 1 | 0 | 84 |
| **Brown betty** | 39 | 1 average serving | 10 | 2 | med | 260 |
| **Brown sauce** | 4 | 1 level tbsp | 0 | trace | low | 15 |
| **Brownie**, chocolate | 63 | 1 brownie | 11 | 5 | med | 368 |
| **Brunswick stew** | 46 | 1 average serving | 12 | 39 | high | 444 |
| **Brussels sprouts**, steamed or boiled | 3 | 3 heaped tbsp | 1 | 3 | high | 35 |
| Brussels sprouts, with chestnuts | 20 | 3 heaped tbsp | 43 | 2 | high | 176 |
| **Bubble and squeak** | 7 | 1 average serving | 18 | 3 | high | 240 |
| **Bucatini** (long macaroni), dried, boiled | 51 | 1 average serving | 2 | 8 | med | 239 |

| Food | Carbo-hydrate g | Portion size | Fat g | Protein g | Fibre | kCalories per portion |
|---|---|---|---|---|---|---|
| Bucatini, fresh, boiled | 57 | 1 average serving | 2 | 11 | med | 301 |
| **Buck rarebit** | 22 | 1 slice | 19 | 17 | low | 312 |
| **Buckling**, smoked | 0 | 1 med fish | 44 | 26 | 0 | 520 |
| **Buckwheat noodles**, boiled | 48 | 1 average serving | trace | 11 | low | 228 |
| **Buckwheat pancakes** | 6 | 1 pancake | 2 | 2 | low | 45 |
| **Bulgar** (cracked wheat), cooked | 29 | 3 heaped tbsp | 4 | 6 | med | 177 |
| **Buns** See individual flavours, e.g. Currant bun | | | | | | |
| **Burger bun** | 24 | 1 bun | 2 | 4 | low | 132 |
| **Burgers** See individual varieties, e.g. Hamburger | | | | | | |
| **Burritos**, with beans and cheese | 55 | 2 burritos | 12 | 15 | med | 377 |
| Burritos, with beef, beans and cheese | 40 | 2 burritos | 13 | 15 | med | 331 |
| **Butter** | trace | 25 g/1 oz/2 tbsp | 20 | trace | 0 | 184 |
| Butter | trace | 1 small knob | 8 | trace | 0 | 74 |
| **Butter** (lima) **beans**, canned, drained | 13 | 3 heaped tbsp | trace | 6 | high | 77 |
| Butter beans, dried, soaked and cooked | 18 | 3 heaped tbsp | 1 | 7 | high | 103 |
| **Butter pecan ice cream** | 12 | 1 scoop | 4 | 2 | low | 91 |
| **Butter puffs** | 6 | 1 biscuit | 3 | 1 | low | 54 |

| Food | Carbo-hydrate g | Portion size | Fat g | Protein g | Fibre | kCalories per portion |
|---|---|---|---|---|---|---|
| **Butter sauce** | 8 | 5 level tbsp | 8 | 3 | low | 112 |
| **Butter shortcake biscuits** (cookies) | 7 | 1 biscuit | 2 | 1 | low | 50 |
| **Butter/vegetable fat spread** | trace | 25 g/1 oz/2 tbsp | 18 | trace | 0 | 165 |
| Butter/vegetable fat spread | trace | 1 small knob | 7 | trace | 0 | 66 |
| **Buttercream icing** (frosting) | 9 | 1 level tbsp | 3 | trace | 0 | 40 |
| **Butterfly cakes** | 26 | 1 individual cake | 15 | 2 | low | 245 |
| **Butterfly prawns** (jumbo shrimp), fried (sautéed), in breadcrumbs | 35 | 6 prawns | 23 | 16 | low | 405 |
| **Buttermilk** | 8 | 150 ml/¼ pt | trace | 6 | 0 | 60 |
| **Butternut squash,** steamed or boiled | 2 | ½ med squash | trace | trace | low | 9 |
| **Butterscotch** | 5 | 1 piece | trace | trace | 0 | 24 |
| **Butterscotch sauce** | 32 | 2 level tbsp | 2 | 1 | low | 145 |
| **Butterscotch tart** | 57 | 1 average slice | 23 | 10 | low | 531 |

| Food | Carbo-hydrate g | Portion size | Fat g | Protein g | Fibre | kCalories per portion |
|---|---|---|---|---|---|---|
| **Cabbage**, green, steamed or boiled | 2 | 3 heaped tbsp | trace | 1 | med | 16 |
| Cabbage, red/white, pickled | **trace** | 1 level tbsp | 0 | trace | med | 3 |
| Cabbage, red/white, raw | 5 | 3 heaped tbsp | trace | 1 | med | 27 |
| Cabbage leaves, stuffed | 19 | 2 leaves | 9 | 18 | high | 221 |
| **Cabinet pudding** | 36 | 1 average serving | 2 | 3 | med | 233 |
| **Caerphilly cheese** | **trace** | 1 small wedge | 8 | 6 | 0 | 94 |
| **Caesar salad** | 6 | 1 average serving | 13 | 17 | med | 207 |
| **Café noir biscuits** (cookies) | 8 | 1 biscuit | trace | trace | low | 39 |
| **Caffé latte** | 10 | 1 med cup | 8 | 6 | 0 | 133 |
| **Cajun chicken** | 33 | 1 average serving | 9 | 40 | med | 366 |
| **Cake**, chocolate | 58 | 1 average slice | 14 | 5 . | low | 384 |
| Cake, light fruit | 58 | 1 average slice | 13 | 5 | med | 354 |
| Cake, plain | 58 | 1 average slice | 17 | 5 | low | 393 |
| Cake, rich fruit | 60 | 1 average slice | 11 | 4 | med | 341 |
| *See also Sponge cake and individual lavours, e.g. Coffee cake* | | | | | | |
| **Calabrese**, steamed or boiled | 2 | 4 medium florets | 1 | 4 | med | 33 |
| **Calamari rings**, fried (sautéed), in batter | 19 | 1 average serving | 12 | 14 | low | 235 |
| **Calippo** ice lolly, any flavour | 26 | 1 lolly | trace | trace | 0 | 105 |

| Food | Carbo-hydrate g | Portion size | Fat g | Protein g | Fibre | kCalories per portion |
|---|---|---|---|---|---|---|
| **Calvados** | trace | 1 single measure | 0 | trace | 0 | 55 |
| **Calves' liver,** braised | 3 | 3 med slices | 7 | 22 | low | 165 |
| Calves' liver, fried (sautéed), in seasoned flour | 7 | 3 med slices | 13 | 27 | 0 | 254 |
| **Calypso coffee** | 7 | 1 wine glass | 14 | 1 | 0 | 218 |
| **Calzone** | 50 | 1 individual pie | 24 | 18 | med | 470 |
| **Cambozola cheese** | trace | 1 small wedge | 10 | 4 | 0 | 106 |
| **Camembert cheese** | trace | 1 small wedge | 6 | 5 | 0 | 74 |
| **Camp coffee,** made with semi-skimmed milk | 15 | 1 mug | 4 | 8 | 0 | 125 |
| Camp coffee, made with skimmed milk | 15 | 1 mug | trace | 8 | 0 | 93 |
| **Candied fruits** *See* Glacé fruits | | | | | | |
| **Candied peel** *See* Mixed peel | | | | | | |
| **Candy** *See individual varieties, e.g.* Chocolate brazils, Lemon drops | | | | | | |
| **Candy floss** | 26 | 1 stick | 0 | trace | 0 | 100 |
| **Cannellini beans,** canned, drained | 22 | 3 heaped tbsp | 1 | 8 | high | 101 |
| Cannellini beans, dried, soaked and cooked | 17 | 3 heaped tbsp | trace | 8 | high | 103 |

| Food | Carbo-hydrate g | Portion size | Fat g | Protein g | Fibre | kCalories per portion |
|---|---|---|---|---|---|---|
| **Cannelloni**, filled with meat | **24** | 2 tubes | 17 | 12 | med | 298 |
| Cannelloni, filled with spinach and ricotta | **17** | 2 tubes | 16 | 9 | med | 250 |
| **Cantal cheese** | trace | 1 small wedge | 8 | 6 | 0 | 101 |
| **Canteloupe melon** | **13** | ½ melon | trace | 2 | med | 57 |
| **Cape gooseberries** | trace | 1 fruit | trace | trace | low | 3 |
| **Cappellini** (pasta strands), dried, boiled | **51** | 1 average serving | 2 | 8 | med | 239 |
| Cappellini, fresh, boiled | **57** | 1 average serving | 2 | 11 | med | 301 |
| **Caper sauce**, made with semi-skimmed milk | **10** | 5 level tbsp | 6 | 4 | low | 103 |
| Caper sauce, made with skimmed milk | **10** | 5 level tbsp | 5 | 4 | low | 93 |
| **Capercaillie, roast** | **0** | ¼ bird | 5 | 31 | 0 | 173 |
| **Capers**, pickled | **2** | 1 level tbsp | 0 | trace | low | 7 |
| **Capon**, roast, with skin | **0** | 3 med slices | 14 | 23 | 0 | 216 |
| Capon, roast, without skin | **0** | 3 med slices | 5 | 25 | 0 | 148 |
| **Caponata** | **15** | 1 average slice | 1 | 3 | med | 85 |
| **Cappelletti** (stuffed pasta), dried, all stuffings | **45** | 1 average serving | 6 | 9 | med | 291 (average) |
| Cappelletti, fresh, all stuffings | **40** | 1 average serving | 4 | 9 | med | 229 (average) |
| **Cappuccino** | **7** | 1 med cup | 6 | 2 | 0 | 101 |

| Food | Carbo-hydrate g | Portion size | Fat g | Protein g | Fibre | kCalories per portion |
|------|------|------|------|------|------|------|
| **Capsicum** *See* Pepper | | | | | | |
| **Caramac** chocolate bar | 16 | 1 standard bar | 11 | 2 | 0 | 170 |
| **Caramel ice cream** | 12 | 1 scoop | 4 | 2 | low | 89 |
| **Caramel shortcake** | 20 | 1 slice | 9 | 1 | low | 171 |
| **Caramel toffees** | 6 | 1 toffee | 1 | trace | 0 | 29 |
| **Caramel wafers** | 17 | 1 standard bar | 5 | 1 | low | 113 |
| **Carbonara pasta sauce** | 5 | ¼ jar | 20 | 2 | 0 | 163 |
| **Carob bar** | 49 | 1 standard bar | 27 | 7 | high | 470 |
| **Carpaccio of beef** | 0 | 2 thin slices | 2 | 10 | 0 | 61 |
| **Carrot** | 8 | 1 large carrot | trace | 1 | med | 35 |
| **Carrot and orange soup** | 12 | 2 ladlefuls | 3 | 1 | med | 78 |
| **Carrot cake** | 47 | 1 average slice | 7 | 3 | med | 260 |
| **Carrot juice** | 6 | 1 small glass | trace | trace | 0 | 24 |
| **Carrots,** honey-glazed | 9 | 3 heaped tbsp | trace | 1 | med | 39 |
| Carrots, steamed or boiled | 5 | 3 heaped tbsp | trace | 1 | med | 24 |
| **Cashew nuts,** fresh | 4 | 25 g/1 oz/¼ cup | 12 | 5 | high | 143 |
| Cashew nuts, roasted | 3 | 1 small handful | 8 | 3 | high | 92 |
| **Cassata** | 14 | 1 average serving | 23 | 3 | low | 227 |
| **Cassava,** baked | 80 | 5 med slices | trace | 2 | high | 310 |
| Cassava, boiled | 33 | 5 med slices | trace | trace | high | 130 |
| **Cassoulet** | 38 | 1 average serving | 13 | 21 | high | 341 |
| **Castle pudding** | 36 | 1 ind pudding | 2 | 3 | med | 233 |

| Food | Carbo-hydrate g | Portion size | Fat g | Protein g | Fibre | kCalories per portion |
|---|---|---|---|---|---|---|
| **Catfish**, fried (sautéed), in breadcrumbs | 9 | 1 piece of fillet | 15 | 21 | low | 265 |
| Catfish, grilled (broiled) | 0 | 1 piece of fillet | 2 | 27 | 0 | 217 |
| Catfish, steamed or poached | 0 | 1 piece of fillet | 2 | 31 | 0 | 141 |
| **Catsup** See Ketchup | | | | | | |
| **Cauliflower** | 3 | 4 medium florets | 1 | 4 | med | 34 |
| Cauliflower, in white sauce, made with semi-skimmed milk | 10 | 3 heaped tbsp | 7 | 6 | med | 124 |
| Cauliflower, in white sauce, made with skimmed milk | 10 | 3 heaped tbsp | 6 | 6 | med | 114 |
| Cauliflower, steamed or boiled | 2 | 4 medium florets | 1 | 3 | med | 28 |
| **Cauliflower bhaji** | 3 | 1 bhaji | 14 | 3 | med | 150 |
| **Cauliflower cheese** | 8 | 1 average serving | 10 | 9 | med | 157 |
| **Cauliflower soup** | 16 | 2 ladlefuls | 5 | 7 | med | 133 |
| **Caviar**, red or black | 1 | 1 level tbsp | 3 | 4 | 0 | 40 |
| **Celeriac** (celery root) | 3 | ¼ small head | trace | 1 | high | 20 |
| Celeriac, steamed or boiled | 2 | 3 heaped tbsp | trace | 1 | high | 15 |
| **Celery** | trace | 1 stick | trace | trace | low | 2 |
| Celery, braised | 1 | 3 heaped tbsp | trace | trace | med | 8 |
| **Celery root** See Celeriac | | | | | | |
| **Celery soup**, cream of, canned | 7 | 2 ladlefuls | 6 | 2 | low | 86 |

| Food | Carbo-hydrate g | Portion size | Fat g | Protein g | Fibre | kCalories per portion |
|---|---|---|---|---|---|---|
| Celery soup, home-made | 11 | 2 ladlefuls | 2 | 5 | med | 82 |
| Celery soup, packet | 8 | 2 ladlefuls | 2 | 2 | low | 50 |
| Cellophane noodles, boiled | 57 | 1 average serving | trace | 2 | low | 251 |
| Ceps mushrooms, stewed | trace | 2 tbsp | trace | 1 | low | 6 |
| Cereal bars, chewy all flavours | 21 | 1 bar | 5 | 1 | med | 131 (average) |
| Cereal bars, crunchy, all flavours | 17 | 1 bar | 7 | 2 | med | 146 (average) |
| Cervelat | trace | 1 med slice | 7 | 4 | 0 | 77 |
| Champagne | 2 | 1 wine glass | 0 | trace | 0 | 114 |
| Channa dahl | 10 | 3 heaped tbsp | 6 | 5 | high | 125 |
| Chanterelle mushrooms, stewed | trace | 2 level tbsp | trace | 1 | low | 6 |
| Chantilly cream | trace | 1 level tbsp | 8 | trace | 0 | 72 |
| Chapattis, made with fat | 24 | 1 chapatti | 6 | 4 | med | 164 |
| Chapattis, made without fat | 22 | 1 chapatti | trace | 4 | med | 101 |
| Charentais melon | 13 | ½ melon | trace | 2 | med | 57 |
| Chargrilled chicken sandwiches | 29 | 1 round | 20 | 25 | med | 401 |
| Chargrilled chicken breast | 0 | 1 breast | 4 | 38 | 0 | 192 |
| Charlotte russe | 50 | 1 average serving | 10 | 6 | low | 307 |
| Chasseur sauce | 7 | 5 level tbsp | trace | 1 | 0 | 36 |
| Chaumes cheese | trace | 1 small wedge | 8 | 6 | 0 | 94 |

| Food | Carbo-hydrate g | Portion size | Fat g | Protein g | Fibre | kCalories per portion |
|---|---|---|---|---|---|---|
| **Cheddar cheese** | trace | 1 small wedge | 9 | 6 | 0 | 103 |
| Cheddar cheese, low-fat | trace | 1 small wedge | 4 | 8 | 0 | 65 |
| **Cheddars** | 2 | 1 biscuit (cookie) | 1 | trace | low | 21 |
| **Cheerios**, dry | 18 | 25 g/1 oz/½ cup | 1 | 2 | med | 92 |
| Cheerios, with semi-skimmed milk | 36 | 5 heaped tbsp | 3 | 7 | med | 204 |
| Cheerios, with skimmed milk | 36 | 5 heaped tbsp | 1 | 7 | med | 188 |
| **Cheese**, fresh, soft, full-fat | trace | 1 good spoonful | 8 | 2 | 0 | 78 |
| Cheese, fresh, soft, low-fat | trace | 1 good spoonful | trace | 2 | 0 | 30 |
| Cheese, fresh, soft, med-fat | trace | 1 good spoonful | 4 | 2 | 0 | 44 |
| Cheese, potted | 1 | 1 individual pot | 23 | 12 | 0 | 267 |
| *See also individual names, e.g.* Cheddar | | | | | | |
| **Cheese and bean enchiladas** | 82 | 2 enchiladas | 14 | 28 | high | 547 |
| **Cheese and beef enchiladas** | 60 | 2 enchiladas | 36 | 24 | low | 644 |
| **Cheese and cole-slaw sandwiches** | 36 | 1 round | 28 | 12 | med | 440 |
| **Cheese and ham sandwiches** | 34 | 1 round | 27 | 19 | med | 432 |
| **Cheese and onion quiche** | 24 | 1 large slice | 28 | 14 | med | 396 |
| **Cheese and pickle sandwiches** | 34 | 1 round | 26 | 12 | med | 407 |

| Food | Carbo-hydrate g | Portion size | Fat g | Protein g | Fibre | kCalories per portion |
|---|---|---|---|---|---|---|
| **Cheese and pineapple chunks** | 1 | 1 stick | 2 | 1 | low | 25 |
| **Cheese and tomato pizza**, deep-pan | 30 | 1 large slice | 14 | 15 | med | **300** |
| Cheese and tomato pizza, thin-crust | 25 | 1 large slice | 12 | 9 | med | 235 |
| **Cheese and tomato sandwiches** | 36 | 1 round | 26 | 13 | med | 411 |
| **Cheese fondue** | 8 | 1 average serving | 29 | 30 | 0 | 492 |
| Cheese fondue, with French bread | 62 | 1 serving plus 10 cubes of bread | 31 | 40 | low | 762 |
| **Cheese footballs** | 1 | 1 football | 1 | trace | low | 13 |
| **Cheese melt biscuits** (cookies) | 3 | 1 biscuit | 1 | trace | low | 21 |
| Cheese melt biscuits, mini | 1 | 1 biscuit | trace | trace | low | 6 |
| **Cheese omelette** | trace | 2 eggs | 30 | 21 | 0 | 356 |
| **Cheese on toast** | 21 | 1 slice | 13 | 10 | low | 223 |
| **Cheese pudding** | 24 | 1 average serving | 14 | 17 | low | 292 |
| **Cheese sandwiches** | 34 | 1 round | 26 | 12 | med | 398 |
| **Cheese sauce**, made with semi-skimmed milk | 7 | 5 level tbsp | 10 | 6 | low | 134 |
| Cheese sauce, made with skimmed milk | 7 | 5 level tbsp | 8 | 6 | low | 124 |
| **Cheese scone** (biscuit) | 21 | 1 scone | 9 | 5 | low | 175 |
| Cheese scone, with butter | 21 | 1 scone | 17 | 5 | low | 249 |

| Food | Carbo-hydrate g | Portion size | Fat g | Protein g | Fibre | kCalories per portion |
|---|---|---|---|---|---|---|
| Cheese scone, with low-fat spread | **21** | 1 scone | 13 | 6 | low | 214 |
| **Cheese slice, processed** | **trace** | 1 slice | 5 | 4 | 0 | 65 |
| **Cheese soufflé** | **10** | 1 average serving | 9 | 13 | low | 280 |
| **Cheese soup,** canned | **8** | 2 ladlefuls | 8 | 4 | low | 126 |
| Cheese soup, home-made | **11** | 2 ladlefuls | 3 | 6 | low | 94 |
| **Cheese spread** | **1** | 1 level tbsp | 3 | 2 | 0 | 41 |
| Cheese spread, flavoured | **1** | 1 level tbsp | 3 | 2 | low | 35 |
| Cheese spread, low-fat | **1** | 1 level tbsp | 2 | 2 | 0 | 27 |
| **Cheese straws** | **2** | 1 straw | trace | 1 | low | 28 |
| **Cheeseburger** | **33** | 1 burger in a bun | 11 | 16 | med | 299 |
| **Cheesecake**, plain, cooked | **30** | 1 average slice | 27 | 4 | low | 490 |
| Cheesecake, plain, set | **30** | 1 average slice | 13 | 5 | low | 272 |
| Cheesecake, with fruit topping | **41** | 1 average slice | 13 | 7 | low | 302 |
| *See also individual flavours, e.g. Chocolate cheesecake* | | | | | | |
| **Cheeselets** | **16** | 1 small bag | 8 | 3 | med | 147 |
| **Chelsea bun** | **50** | 1 bun | 12 | 7 | med | 329 |
| **Cherries** | **4** | 10 cherries | trace | trace | low | 20 |

| Food | Carbo-hydrate g | Portion size | Fat g | Protein g | Fibre | kCalories per portion |
|---|---|---|---|---|---|---|
| Cherries, canned in natural juice | 13 | 3 heaped tbsp | trace | trace | low | 51 |
| Cherries, canned in syrup | 18 | 3 heaped tbsp | trace | trace | low | 71 |
| Cherries, glacé (candied) | 4 | 1 cherry | trace | trace | low | 13 |
| Cherries, in brandy/ kirsch | 18 | 3 heaped tbsp | trace | trace | low | 126 |
| Cherries, maraschino | 3 | 1 cherry | trace | trace | low | 12 |
| **Cherry bakewells** | 32 | 1 individual cake | 8 | 2 | low | 206 |
| **Cherry brandy** | 8 | 1 single measure | 0 | trace | 0 | 64 |
| **Cherry cheesecake** | 41 | 1 average slice | 13 | 7 | low | 302 |
| **Cherry compôte** | 20 | 3 heaped tbsp | trace | 1 | low | 78 |
| **Cherry genoa cake** | 51 | 1 average slice | 12 | 4 | med | 334 |
| **Cherry pie** | 40 | 1 average slice | 13 | 3 | med | 282 |
| **Cherry pie filling** | 21 | ¼ large can | trace | trace | low | 82 |
| **Cherryade** | 21 | 1 tumbler | trace | trace | 0 | 18 |
| **Cheshire cheese** | trace | 1 small wedge | 8 | 6 | 0 | 94 |
| **Chestnut purée**, sweetened | 10 | 1 level tbsp | trace | trace | med | 45 |
| Chestnut purée, unsweetened | 5 | 1 level tbsp | trace | trace | med | 25 |
| **Chestnut stuffing** | 4 | 1 average serving | 4 | 1 | med | 58 |
| **Chestnuts** | 4 | 1 nut | trace | trace | high | 18 |
| Chestnuts, peeled and cooked | 14 | 5 nuts | trace | 1 | high | 65 |
| Chestnuts, roasted in shells | 4 | 1 nut | trace | trace | high | 21 |
| **Chèvre cheese** | trace | 1 small wedge | 7 | 5 | 0 | 80 |

| Food | Carbo-hydrate g | Portion size | Fat g | Protein g | Fibre | kCalories per portion |
|---|---|---|---|---|---|---|
| **Chewy cereal bars**, all flavours | 21 | 1 bar | 5 | 1 | med | 131 (average) |
| **Chick pea dahl** | 10 | 3 heaped tbsp | 6 | 5 | high | 125 |
| **Chick pea goulash** | 36 | 1 average serving | 15 | 12 | high | 338 |
| **Chick peas** (garbanzos), canned, drained | 16 | 3 heaped tbsp | 3 | 7 | high | 115 |
| Chick peas, dried, soaked and boiled | 18 | 3 heaped tbsp | 2 | 8 | high | 121 |
| **Chicken**, breast, cooked, sliced | 0 | 1 med slice | 1 | 7 | 0 | 35 |
| Chicken, breast, grilled (broiled) | 0 | 1 med breast | 6 | 40 | 0 | 213 |
| Chicken, breast, poached or steamed | 0 | 1 med breast | 7 | 44 | 0 | 244 |
| Chicken, breast, smoked | trace | 1 med slice | 1 | 2 | 0 | 23 |
| Chicken, breast portion, fried (sautéed), in breadcrumbs | 22 | ¼ small chicken | 19 | 27 | low | 363 |
| Chicken, drumstick, barbecued | 2 | 1 drumstick | 4 | 16 | 0 | 103 |
| Chicken, drumstick, roast | 0 | 1 drumstick | 3 | 15 | 0 | 92 |
| Chicken, fried | 19 | 2 pieces | 29 | 36 | low | 494 |
| Chicken, jerk | 15 | 1 average serving | 8 | 32 | high | 256 |
| Chicken, leg portion barbecued | 1 | ¼ small chicken | 10 | 46 | 0 | 287 |
| Chicken, leg portion, grilled | 0 | ¼ small chicken | 10 | 46 | 0 | 274 |

| Food | Carbo-hydrate g | Portion size | Fat g | Protein g | Fibre | kCalories per portion |
|---|---|---|---|---|---|---|
| Chicken, leg portion, roast | 0 | ¼ small chicken | 10 | 46 | 0 | 276 |
| Chicken, lemon | 3 | 1 medium breast | 13 | 58 | 0 | 356 |
| Chicken, minced (ground), stewed | 0 | 1 average serving | 7 | 29 | 0 | 183 |
| Chicken, roast, with skin | 0 | 3 medium slices | 14 | 23 | 0 | 216 |
| Chicken, roast, without skin | 0 | 3 medium slices | 5 | 25 | 0 | 148 |
| Chicken, steamed | 0 | ¼ small chicken | 7 | 29 | low | 197 |
| Chicken, sweet and sour | 32 | 1 average serving | 2 | 6 | high | 165 |
| Chicken, tandoori | 4 | ¼ small chicken | 19 | 47 | trace | 375 |
| Chicken, thai, with noodles | 59 | 1 serving | 15 | 34 | high | 506 |
| Chicken, wing portion, grilled (broiled) | 0 | ¼ small chicken | 9 | 36 | 0 | 220 |
| Chicken, wing portion, roast | 0 | ¼ small chicken | 9 | 36 | 0 | 222 |
| Chicken, wings, barbecued, Chinese-style | 3 | 1 wing | 2 | 9 | 0 | 70 |
| **Chicken à la king** | 20 | 1 average serving | 9 | 23 | med | 255 |
| **Chicken and almond soup**, canned | 9 | 2 ladlefuls | 14 | 5 | low | 180 |
| **Chicken and sweetcorn (corn) chowder**, home-made | 16 | 2 ladlefuls | 3 | 25 | med | 183 |

| Food | Carbo-hydrate g | Portion size | Fat g | Protein g | Fibre | kCalories per portion |
|------|---------------|--------------|-------|-----------|-------|----------------------|
| Chicken and sweetcorn soup, canned | 12 | 2 ladlefuls | 2 | 3 | low | 84 |
| Chicken and sweetcorn soup, instant | 16 | 1 mug | 6 | 1 | low | 119 |
| **Chicken and ham paste** | trace | 1 level tbsp | 4 | 4 | 0 | 56 |
| **Chicken and ham pie**, cold | 32 | 1 average slice | 22 | 12 | low | 380 |
| **Chicken and mush-room casserole** | 29 | 1 average serving | 16 | 39 | low | 413 |
| **Chicken and mush-room chowder** | 17 | 2 ladlefuls | 10 | 7 | low | 192 |
| **Chicken and mushroom pie** | 17 | 1 individual pie | 12 | 16 | low | 246 |
| **Chicken and mushroom soup**, canned | 7 | 2 ladlefuls | 4 | 2 | low | 76 |
| Chicken and mush-room soup, instant | 9 | 1 mug | 2 | 1 | low | 58 |
| **Chicken and rice soup**, canned | 15 | 2 ladlefuls | 2 | 1 | low | 82 |
| Chicken and rice soup, home-made | 13 | 2 ladlefuls | 3 | 12 | low | 127 |
| **Chicken and tarragon soup**, home-made | 9 | 2 ladlefuls | 8 | 3 | low | 116 |
| **Chicken and vegetable soup**, canned | 12 | 2 ladlefuls | 2 | 4 | med | **82** |

| Food | Carbo-hydrate g | Portion size | Fat g | Protein g | Fibre | kCalories per portion |
|---|---|---|---|---|---|---|
| Chicken and vegetable soup, home-made | 19 | 2 ladlefuls | 5 | 12 | high | 165 |
| Chicken and vegetable stir-fry | 39 | 1 average serving | 7 | 22 | high | 270 |
| Chicken broth | 11 | 2 ladlefuls | 2 | 2 | low | 64 |
| Chicken burger in a bun, home-made, with relish | 32 | 1 burger in a bun | 10 | 38 | med | 366 |
| Chicken burger sandwich | 54 | 1 burger | 43 | 26 | med | 710 |
| Chicken byriani | 75 | 1 average serving | 38 | 18 | med | 782 |
| Chicken cacciatore | 36 | 1 average serving | 4 | 22 | high | 265 |
| Chicken casserole | 29 | 1 average serving | 12 | 38 | high | 374 |
| Chicken chasseur | 67 | 1 average serving | 7 | 27 | med | 440 |
| Chicken chop suey | 34 | 1 average serving | 6 | 23 | med | 295 |
| Chicken chow mein | 28 | 1 average serving | 5 | 22 | high | 337 |
| Chicken cordon bleu | 15 | 1 average serving | 20 | 25 | low | 344 |
| Chicken curry, home-made | 9 | 1 average serving | 51 | 31 | med | 615 |
| Chicken curry, home-made, with rice | 65 | 1 average serving | 53 | 36 | med | 863 |
| Chicken curry, retail | 16 | 1 average serving | 27 | 36 | med | 447 |
| Chicken curry, retail, with rice | 68 | 1 average serving | 26 | 37 | high | 691 |
| Chicken enchiladas | 66 | 2 enchiladas | 9 | 32 | high | 566 |
| Chicken fajitas | 34 | 2 fajitas | 6 | 16 | low | 258 |
| Chicken fingers | 2 | 1 finger | 1 | 4 | low | 27 |
| Chicken fricassée | 6 | 1 average serving | 16 | 28 | med | 280 |

| Food | Carbo-hydrate g | Portion size | Fat g | Protein g | Fibre | kCalories per portion |
|---|---|---|---|---|---|---|
| **Chicken galantine** | 9 | 1 average slice | 14 | 26 | med | 268 |
| **Chicken goujons** | 12 | 6 goujons | 3 | 24 | low | 162 |
| **Chicken in black bean sauce** | 10 | 1 average serving | 6 | 29 | med | 221 |
| **Chicken jalfrezi** | 70 | 1 average serving | 12 | 26 | high | 490 |
| **Chicken kiev** | 22 | 1 med breast | 31 | 28 | low | 473 |
| **Chicken korma** | 16 | 1 average serving | 21 | 54 | med | 460 |
| **Chicken liver pâté** | 1 | 1 average serving | 14 | 6 | 0 | 158 |
| **Chicken liver pâté,** with toast and butter | 37 | 1 serving plus 2 slices of toast | 32 | 13 | med | 468 |
| **Chicken liver risotto** | 89 | 1 average serving | 27 | 13 | low | 590 |
| **Chicken livers**, fried (sautéed) | 3 | 1 average serving | 11 | 21 | 0 | 194 |
| **Chicken marsala** | 2 | 1 average serving | 5 | 27 | low | 284 |
| **Chicken maryland** | 30 | ¼ small chicken | 25 | 36 | low | 484 |
| **Chicken mayonnaise sandwiches** | 34 | 1 round | 41 | 12 | med | 458 |
| **Chicken noodle soup**, canned | 8 | 2 ladlefuls | trace | 3 | low | 50 |
| Chicken noodle soup, home-made | 17 | 2 ladlefuls | 4 | 10 | low | 145 |
| Chicken noodle soup, packet | 7 | 2 ladlefuls | 1 | 2 | low | 40 |
| **Chicken nuggets** | 11 | 6 nuggets | 15 | 19 | med | 253 |
| **Chicken omelette** | trace | 2 eggs | 23 | 21 | 0 | 293 |
| **Chicken paprika** | 6 | 1 average serving | 7 | 31 | low | 194 |
| **Chicken paste** | trace | 1 level tbsp | 3 | 2 | 0 | 35 |

| Food | Carbo-hydrate g | Portion size | Fat g | Protein g | Fibre | kCalories per portion |
|---|---|---|---|---|---|---|
| **Chicken pie,** individual | 30 | 1 individual pie | 22 | 12 | low | 378 |
| Chicken pie, with puff pastry (paste) | 36 | 1 average serving | 37 | 23 | low | 572 |
| **Chicken pot pie** | 28 | 1 average slice | 39 | 17 | low | 485 |
| **Chicken pot roast with vegetables** | 65 | 1 average serving | 11 | 37 | high | 510 |
| **Chicken ravioli** | 26 | 1 average serving | 1 | 7 | med | 148 |
| **Chicken risotto** | 83 | 1 average serving | 8 | 31 | low | 336 |
| **Chicken roll,** sliced | trace | 1 standard slice | 1 | 3 | 0 | 22 |
| **Chicken salad** | 5 | 1 average serving | 7 | 32 | high | 215 |
| Chicken salad, dressed | 5 | 1 average serving | 19 | 33 | high | 318 |
| **Chicken sandwiches** | 34 | 1 round | 23 | 12 | med | 341 |
| **Chicken satay** | 6 | 1 stick | 5 | 26 | low | 172 |
| **Chicken soup,** cream of, canned | 9 | 2 ladlefuls | 8 | 3 | 0 | 116 |
| Chicken soup, home-made | 7 | 2 ladlefuls | 4 | 12 | 0 | 114 |
| Chicken soup, instant | 11 | 1 mug | 6 | 1 | 0 | 100 |
| Chicken soup, low-fat, canned | 4 | 2 ladlefuls | 2 | 2 | 0 | 44 |
| Chicken soup, packet | 21 | 2 ladlefuls | 5 | 2 | 0 | 128 |
| **Chicken stew with dumplings** | 77 | 1 average serving | 9 | 38 | high | 537 |
| **Chicken suprême** | 8 | 1 breast | 12 | 43 | low | 309 |
| **Chicken tenders** | 17 | 8 pieces | 22 | 22 | low | 350 |
| **Chicken teriyaki** | 52 | 1 average serving | 4 | 19 | high | 317 |
| **Chicken tikka** | 11 | 1 average serving | 17 | 43 | med | 369 |

| Food | Carbo-hydrate g | Portion size | Fat g | Protein g | Fibre | kCalories per portion |
|---|---|---|---|---|---|---|
| Chicken tikka masala | 44 | 1 average serving | 18 | 38 | high | 490 |
| Chicken véronique | 11 | 1 average serving | 10 | 27 | low | 254 |
| Chicken vindaloo | 7 | 1 average serving | 40 | 48 | med | 572 |
| Chicory (Belgian endive) | trace | 1 head | 2 | 2 | low | 18 |
| Chicory, braised | 2 | 1 head | 2 | 3 | low | 38 |
| Chilli beans | 52 | 1 average serving | 2 | 15 | high | 247 |
| Chilli con carne | 17 | 1 average serving | 17 | 22 | high | 302 |
| Chilli dog | 29 | 1 dog in a bun | 7 | 7 | low | 204 |
| Chilli salsa | 4 | 1 level tbsp | trace | trace | low | 18 |
| Chilli sauce | 3 | 1 level tbsp | trace | trace | low | 15 |
| Chinese egg noodles, cooked | 26 | 1 average serving | 1 | 4 | med | 124 |
| Chinese leaves (stem lettuce) | 1 | 1 average serving | 0 | 1 | low | 11 |
| Chinese pork spare ribs | 13 | 2 ribs | 17 | 25 | low | 310 |
| Chipolata sausages, fried (sautéed) | 2 | 1 sausage | 5 | 3 | low | 61 |
| Chipolata sausages, grilled (broiled) | 2 | 1 sausage | 5 | 3 | low | 58 |
| Chips (fries), chip-shop | 49 | 1 average serving | 20 | 5 | high | 394 |
| Chips, crinkle-cut, frozen, deep-fried | 55 | 1 average serving | 27 | 6 | high | 478 |
| Chips, home-made, deep-fried | 50 | 1 average serving | 11 | 6 | high | 312 |
| Chips, microwave | 32 | 1 small box | 10 | 4 | high | 221 |

| Food | Carbo-hydrate g | Portion size | Fat g | Protein g | Fibre | kCalories per portion |
|---|---|---|---|---|---|---|
| Chips, oven, frozen, baked | 49 | 1 average serving | 7 | 5 | high | 267 |
| Chips, straight-cut, frozen, deep-fried | 53 | 1 average serving | 16 | 6 | high | 450 |
| Chips, thin-cut | 56 | 1 average serving | 26 | 5 | high | 462 |
| *See also* French fries | | | | | | |
| **Choc ice**, any chocolate | 18 | 1 ice cream | 11 | 2 | low | 180 |
| **Choco corn flakes**, dry | 21 | 25 g/1 oz/½ cup | 1 | 1 | low | 95 |
| Choco corn flakes, with semi-skimmed milk | 35 | 5 heaped tbsp | 3 | 6 | low | 209 |
| Choco corn flakes, with skimmed milk | 35 | 5 heaped tbsp | 1 | 6 | low | 193 |
| **Chocolate**, milk | 28 | 1 standard bar | 14 | 4 | 0 | 255 |
| Chocolate, plain (semi-sweet) | 30 | 1 standard bar | 13 | 2 | 0 | 250 |
| Chocolate, white | 11 | 1 standard bar | 6 | 2 | 0 | 109 |
| Chocolate, with fruit and nut | 27 | 1 standard bar | 12 | 4 | 0 | 240 |
| Chocolate, with whole nuts | 24 | 1 standard bar | 17 | 5 | 0 | 270 |
| **Chocolate and walnut brownies** | 40 | 1 brownie | 37 | 7 | med | 505 |
| **Chocolate biscuits (cookies)**, full-coated | 17 | 1 biscuit | 7 | 1 | low | 131 |
| Chocolate biscuits, half-coated | 11 | 1 biscuit | 4 | 1 | low | 84 |
| **Chocolate brazils** | 3 | 1 sweet (candy) | 4 | 1 | high | 49 |

| Food | Carbo-hydrate g | Portion size | Fat g | Protein g | Fibre | kCalories per portion |
|---|---|---|---|---|---|---|
| **Chocolate brownies** | 63 | 1 brownie | 11 | 5 | med | 368 |
| **Chocolate buttons** | 19 | 1 small packet | 10 | 3 | 0 | 175 |
| **Chocolate cake,** chocolate-coated | 41 | 1 average slice | 10 | 3 | low | 268 |
| Chocolate cake, filled with butter cream | 35 | 1 average slice | 10 | 3 | low | 235 |
| **Chocolate caramels** | 6 | 1 sweet (candy) | trace | trace | low | 25 |
| **Chocolate cheesecake** | 34 | 1 average slice | 11 | 12 | low | 271 |
| **Chocolate chip chewy cereal bar** | 17 | 1 bar | 4 | 1 | low | 112 |
| **Chocolate chip cookies** | 8 | 1 cookie | 1 | trace | low | 45 |
| **Chocolate chip ice cream** | 12 | 1 scoop | 4 | 2 | low | 91 |
| **Chocolate chip muffin** | 51 | 1 muffin | 22 | 5 | low | 397 |
| **Chocolate corn pops**, dry | 20 | 25 g/1 oz/½ cup | 1 | 1 | low | 97 |
| Chocolate corn pops, with semi-skimmed milk | 38 | 5 heaped tbsp | 4 | 6 | low | 213 |
| Chocolate corn pops, with skimmed milk | 38 | 5 heaped tbsp | 2 | 6 | low | 197 |
| **Chocolate cream biscuits** (cookies) | 9 | 1 biscuit | 3 | 1 | low | 63 |
| **Chocolate cream pie** | 38 | 1 average slice | 22 | 3 | low | 343 |
| **Chocolate crispix,** dry | 21 | 25 g/1 oz/½ cup | 1 | 1 | low | 90 |

| Food | Carbo-hydrate g | Portion size | Fat g | Protein g | Fibre | kCalories per portion |
|---|---|---|---|---|---|---|
| Chocolate crispix, with semi-skimmed milk | 40 | 5 heaped tbsp | 3 | 6 | low | 201 |
| Chocolate crispix, with skimmed milk | 40 | 5 heaped tbsp | 1 | 6 | low | 185 |
| **Chocolate custard**, canned | 11 | ¼ large can | 2 | 2 | low | 71 |
| **Chocolate dessert** | 19 | 1 individual pot | 5 | 2 | low | 136 |
| Chocolate dessert, with cream | 24 | 1 individual pot | 12 | 4 | low | 225 |
| **Chocolate digestives** (graham crackers) | 11 | 1 biscuit (cookie) | 4 | 1 | med | 88 |
| **Chocolate éclair toffees** | 7 | 1 toffee | 2 | trace | low | 48 |
| **Chocolate éclair,** filled with cream | 18 | 1 éclair | 21 | 4 | low | 277 |
| Chocolate éclair, filled with custard | 24 | 1 éclair | 16 | 6 | low | 262 |
| **Chocolate finger biscuits** (cookies) | 5 | 1 biscuit | 2 | trace | low | 38 |
| **Chocolate fudge** | 13 | 1 piece | 1 | trace | low | 65 |
| **Chocolate fudge cake** | 70 | 1 average slice | 14 | 5 | low | 420 |
| **Chocolate fudge fingers** | 22 | 1 finger | 5 | 1 | 0 | 135 |
| **Chocolate fudge icing** (frosting) | 9 | 1 level tbsp | 1 | trace | low | 77 |
| **Chocolate ginger** | 7 | 1 piece | trace | trace | low | 30 |
| **Chocolate ice cream** | 12 | 1 scoop | 4 | 2 | low | 89 |

| Food | Carbo-hydrate g | Portion size | Fat g | Protein g | Fibre | kCalories per portion |
|---|---|---|---|---|---|---|
| **Chocolate layer cake** | 58 | 1 average slice | 14 | 5 | low | 384 |
| **Chocolate mini roll** | 16 | 1 roll | 5 | 1 | low | 119 |
| **Chocolate mint creams** | 8 | 1 mint | 1 | trace | 0 | 39 |
| **Chocolate mousse** | 20 | 1 individual pot | 5 | 4 | 0 | 139 |
| Chocolate mousse, low-calorie | 10 | 1 individual pot | 3 | 0 | 0 | 88 |
| **Chocolate nut sundae** | 52 | 1 sundae | 23 | 4 | low | 417 |
| **Chocolate peanuts** | 19 | 1 small packet | 13 | 5 | med | 200 |
| **Chocolate pot** | 19 | 1 individual pot | 5 | 2 | low | 136 |
| **Chocolate profiteroles** | 33 | 1 average serving | 24 | 6 | med | 373 |
| **Chocolate pudding** | 45 | 1 average serving | 16 | 6 | med | 340 |
| **Chocolate raisins** | 32 | 1 small packet | 7 | 2 | high | 185 |
| **Chocolate ripple ice-cream** | 12 | 1 scoop | 4 | 2 | low | 89 |
| **Chocolate roulade** | 20 | 1 average serving | 12 | 4 | 0 | 206 |
| **Chocolate sauce,** for ice cream | 29 | 2 level tbsp | 6 | 5 | low | 192 |
| Chocolate sauce, made with semi-skimmed milk | 14 | 5 level tbsp | 5 | 3 | low | 112 |
| Chocolate sauce, made with skimmed milk | 14 | 5 level tbsp | 4 | 3 | low | 102 |
| **Chocolate shreddies**, dry | 20 | 25 g/1 oz/½ cup | trace | 2 | med | 91 |

| Food | Carbo-hydrate g | Portion size | Fat g | Protein g | Fibre | kCalories per portion |
|------|-----------------|--------------|-------|-----------|-------|-----------------------|
| Chocolate shreddies, with semi-skimmed milk | 42 | 5 heaped tbsp | 3 | 8 | high | 224 |
| Chocolate shreddies, with skimmed milk | 42 | 5 heaped tbsp | 1 | 8 | high | 208 |
| Chocolate soufflé | 17 | 1 average serving | 1 | 7 | low | 103 |
| Chocolate soya ice dessert | 5 | 1 scoop | 3 | 1 | 0 | 52 |
| Chocolate spread, all types | 9 | 1 level tbsp | 5 | 1 | low | 82 (average) |
| Chocolate spread, with peanut butter | 5 | 1 level tbsp | 7 | 2 | med | 89 |
| Chocolate wafer bar | 13 | 1 standard bar | 6 | 1 | 0 | 115 |
| Chocolates, assorted, filled | 7 | 1 chocolate | 2 | trace | 0 | 46 (average) |
| Chorizo sausage | 1 | 1 small sausage | 23 | 14 | 0 | 273 |
| Choux buns, filled with cream | 8 | 1 bun | 21 | 4 | low | 237 |
| Choux buns, filled with custard | 27 | 1 bun | 17 | 7 | low | 293 |
| Christmas cake, with marzipan and royal icing (frosting) | 63 | 1 average slice | 11 | 4 | med | 356 |
| Christmas pudding | 49 | 1 average serving | 10 | 5 | med | 291 |
| Ciabatta bread | 26 | 1 med slice | trace | 4 | med | 125 |
| Cider, dry | 8 | 1 small | 0 | trace | 0 | 108 |
| Cider, med-sweet | 13 | 1 small | 0 | trace | 0 | 126 |
| Cider, vintage | 22 | 1 small | 0 | trace | 0 | 303 |
| Cider cup | 17 | 1 wine glass | 0 | trace | 0 | 62 |

| Food | Carbo-hydrate g | Portion size | Fat g | Protein g | Fibre | kCalories per portion |
|---|---|---|---|---|---|---|
| **Cigarettes russes** | 6 | 1 biscuit (cookie) | 3 | 1 | low | 56 |
| **Cinnamon danish** pastries | 52 | 1 pastry | 18 | 6 | med | 270 |
| **Cinnamon grahams,** dry | 19 | 25 g/1 oz/½ cup | 2 | 1 | med | 102 |
| Cinnamon grahams, with semi-skimmed milk | 29 | 3 heaped tbsp | 5 | 5 | med | 182 |
| Cinnamon grahams, with skimmed milk | 29 | 3 heaped tbsp | 3 | 5 | med | 166 |
| **Clafoutis** | 33 | 1 average serving | 10 | 7 | med | 242 |
| **Clam bisque,** canned | 12 | 2 ladlefuls | 2 | 5 | low | 85 |
| **Clam chowder,** home-made | 17 | 2 ladlefuls | 10 | 22 | med | 253 |
| **Clams,** canned, drained | 2 | ½ medium can | 1 | 9 | 0 | 60 |
| Clams, fresh, shelled, cooked | 4 | 1 average serving | 1 | 15 | 0 | 93 |
| **Classic** chocolate bar | 15 | 1 standard bar | 7 | 1 | low | 125 |
| **Clear conserve** See Jelly, individual flavours, e.g. Redcurrant jelly | | | | | | |
| **Clementine** | 6 | 1 fruit | trace | 1 | med | 28 |
| **Clotted cream** fudge | 14 | 1 square | 3 | trace | 0 | 80 |
| **Club** chocolate bar, all flavours | 16 | 1 bar | 7 | 1 | low | 125 (average) |
| **Clusters,** dry | 17 | 25 g/1 oz/½ cup | 2 | 3 | med | 97 |

| Food | Carbo-hydrate g | Portion size | Fat g | Protein g | Fibre | kCalories per portion |
|------|-----------------|--------------|-------|-----------|-------|----------------------|
| Clusters, with skimmed milk | 26 | 3 heaped tbsp | 3 | 7 | med | 160 |
| Clusters, with semi-skimmed milk | 26 | 3 heaped tbsp | 5 | 7 | med | 176 |
| Cob loaf | 15 | 1 med slice | 1 | 3 | low | 70 |
| Cob nuts, shelled | 1 | 25 g/1 oz/¼ cup | 16 | 3 | med | 162 |
| Cobbler See individual flavours, e.g. Fruit cobbler | | | | | | |
| Coca-cola | 21 | 1 tumbler | 0 | trace | 0 | 78 |
| Coca-cola, diet | 0 | 1 tumbler | 0 | 0 | 0 | 1 |
| Cock-a-leekie soup, home-made | 15 | 2 ladlefuls | 8 | 2 | low | 138 |
| Cockles, fresh, shelled, cooked | trace | 1 average serving | trace | 11 | 0 | 48 |
| Cockles, preserved in vinegar | 1 | 1 average serving | trace | 12 | 0 | 49 |
| Cocktail sauce | 2 | 1 level tbsp | 4 | trace | low | 51 |
| Coco pops, dry | 21 | 25 g/1 oz/½ cup | 1 | 1 | low | 95 |
| Coco pops, with semi-skimmed milk | 27 | 5 heaped tbsp | 3 | 5 | low | 209 |
| Coco pops, with skimmed milk | 27 | 5 heaped tbsp | 1 | 5 | low | 193 |
| Coco pops cereal and milk bar | 14 | 1 bar | 3 | 2 | low | 90 |
| Cocoa, made with semi-skimmed milk and sugar | 17 | 1 mug | 5 | 9 | low | 142 |
| Cocoa, made with skimmed milk and sugar | 17 | 1 mug | 3 | 9 | low | 126 |

| Food | Carbo-hydrate g | Portion size | Fat g | Protein g | Fibre | kCalories per portion |
|------|----------------|--------------|-------|-----------|-------|----------------------|
| Coconut | 13 | ¼ nut | 31 | 3 | high | 330 |
| Coconut, desiccated (shredded) | 1 | 1 level tbsp | 9 | 1 | high | 43 |
| Coconut cake | 20 | 1 average slice | 19 | 3 | low | 175 |
| Coconut ice sweet (candy) bar | 83 | 1 standard bar | 13 | 2 | high | 464 |
| Coconut macaroons | 16 | 1 macaroon | 5 | 1 | med | 117 |
| Coconut pyramid | 42 | 1 pyramid | 6 | 1 | high | 230 |
| Coconut rings/thins | 5 | 1 biscuit (cookie) | 1 | trace | low | 35 |
| Cod, baked | 0 | 1 piece of fillet | 2 | 37 | 0 | 168 |
| Cod, fried (sautéed), in batter | 19 | 1 piece of fillet | 26 | 49 | low | 497 |
| Cod, fried (sautéed), in breadcrumbs | 9 | 1 piece of fillet | 21 | 53 | low | 435 |
| Cod, grilled (broiled) | 0 | 1 piece of fillet | 2 | 36 | 0 | 166 |
| Cod, salt, soaked and cooked | 0 | 1 piece of fillet | 2 | 57 | 0 | 241 |
| Cod, with butter sauce | 9 | 1 steak | 9 | 18 | low | 159 |
| Cod, with cheese sauce | 9 | 1 steak | 6 | 20 | low | 175 |
| Cod, with mushroom sauce | 9 | 1 steak | 8 | 18 | low | 168 |
| Cod, with parsley sauce | 11 | 1 steak | 5 | 19 | low | 170 |
| Cod and prawn pie | 24 | 1 individual pie | 21 | 17 | low | 328 |
| Cod mornay | 23 | 1 steak | 23 | 29 | low | 415 |
| Cod provençal | 9 | 1 average serving | 9 | 39 | med | 273 |

| Food | Carbo-hydrate g | Portion size | Fat g | Protein g | Fibre | kCalories per portion |
|---|---|---|---|---|---|---|
| **Cod roes**, in breadcrumbs, fried (sautéed) | 3 | 1 average serving | 12 | 21 | low | 202 |
| Cod roes, on buttered toast | 10 | 1 serving plus 1 slice of toast | 20 | 20 | low | 307 |
| **Coffee**, black | 1 | 1 mug | trace | trace | 0 | 5 |
| Coffee, espresso | 1 | 1 small cup | trace | trace | 0 | 4 |
| Coffee, white, made with water and semi-skimmed milk | 2 | 1 mug | trace | 1 | 0 | 15 |
| Coffee, white, made with water and skimmed milk | 2 | 1 mug | trace | 1 | 0 | 12 |
| **Coffee and walnut cake** | 34 | 1 average slice | 19 | 7 | med | 344 |
| **Coffee cake** | 34 | 1 average slice | 11 | 5 | low | 258 |
| **Coffee cheesecake** | 30 | 1 average slice | 13 | 5 | low | 272 |
| **Coffee granita** | 11 | 1 average serving | trace | trace | 0 | 44 |
| **Coffee ice cream** | 12 | 1 scoop | 4 | 2 | low | 89 |
| **Coffee mousse** | 20 | 1 average serving | 5 | 4 | 0 | 139 |
| **Coffee roulade** | 20 | 1 average slice | 12 | 4 | 0 | 206 |
| **Coffee streusel cake** | 29 | 1 average slice | 15 | 4 | med | 263 |
| **Coffeemate** | 3 | 1 level tsp | 2 | trace | 0 | 27 |
| Coffeemate, light | 3 | 1 level tsp | 1 | trace | 0 | 21 |
| **Cointreau** | 7 | 1 single measure | 0 | trace | 0 | 78 |
| **Cola** | 21 | 1 tumbler | 0 | trace | 0 | 78 |
| Cola, low-calorie | 0 | 1 tumbler | 0 | 0 | 0 | 1 |
| **Colcannon** | 7 | 1 average serving | 18 | 3 | high | 240 |

| Food | Carbo-hydrate g | Portion size | Fat g | Protein g | Fibre | kCalories per portion |
|---|---|---|---|---|---|---|
| **Coleslaw,** home-made | **13** | 2 good tbsp | 4 | 3 | high | 92 |
| Coleslaw, low-calorie | **2** | 2 good tbsp | 2 | trace | med | 28 |
| Coleslaw, ready-made | **3** | 2 good tbsp | 3 | trace | med | 40 |
| **Coley,** fried (sautéed), in batter | **19** | 1 piece of fillet | 25 | 48 | low | 490 |
| Coley, fried, in breadcrumbs | **9** | 1 piece of fillet | 20 | 52 | low | 428 |
| Coley, poached or steamed | **0** | 1 piece of fillet | 1 | 35 | 0 | 147 |
| **Collard greens** *See* Spring greens | | | | | | |
| **Complan,** savoury, made with water | **24** | 1 mug | 7 | 10 | 0 | 194 |
| Complan, sweet, made with semi-skimmed milk | **34** | 1 mug | 9 | 14 | low | 260 |
| Complan, sweet, made with skimmed milk | **34** | 1 mug | 6 | 14 | low | 240 |
| Complan, sweet, made with water | **27** | 1 mug | 6 | 9 | low | 192 |
| **Conchiglie** (pasta shapes), dried, boiled | **42** | 1 average serving | 1 | 7 | med | 198 |
| Conchiglie, fresh, boiled | **45** | 1 average serving | 2 | 9 | med | 235 |
| **Condensed milk,** skimmed, sweetened | **60** | 100 ml/3½ fl oz/ scant ½ cup | trace | 10 | 0 | 267 |

| Food | Carbo-hydrate g | Portion size | Fat g | Protein g | Fibre | kCalories per portion |
|------|-----------------|--------------|-------|-----------|-------|-----------------------|
| Condensed milk skimmed, unsweetened | 11 | 100 ml/3½ fl oz/ scant ½ cup | trace | 10 | 0 | 80 |
| Condensed milk, whole, sweetened | 55 | 100 ml/3½ fl oz/ scant ½ cup | 10 | 8 | 0 | 333 |
| Condensed milk, whole, unsweetened | 8 | 100 ml/3½ fl oz/ scant ½ cup | 9 | 8 | 0 | 151 |
| **Conger eel**, grilled (broiled) | 0 | 1 steak | 24 | 38 | 0 | 375 |
| **Consommé**, canned | 1 | 2 ladlefuls | trace | 3 | 0 | 14 |
| Consommé, jellied | 2 | 2 ladlefuls | trace | 5 | 0 | 32 |
| **Cookies** *See* Biscuits | | | | | | |
| **Cook-in sauces**, all flavours | 8 | 1 average serving | 1 | 1 | low | 43 (average) |
| **Coq au vin** | 7 | 1 average serving | 29 | 30 | low | 410 |
| **Coquilles st jacques** | 20 | 1 average serving | 10 | 10 | med | 212 |
| **Cordial** *See individual flavours, e.g.* Blackcurrant cordial | | | | | | |
| **Corn chips** | 30 | 1 small bag | 11 | 4 | med | 229 |
| **Corn chowder** | 28 | 2 ladlefuls | 2 | 5 | high | 143 |
| **Corn cobs**, baby, canned, drained | 2 | 4 cobs | trace | 3 | med | 23 |
| Corn cobs, baby, steamed or boiled | 3 | 4 cobs | trace | 2 | med | 24 |
| Corn cobs, baby, stir-fried | 3 | 4 cobs | 5 | 2 | med | 69 |
| **Corn flakes**, dry | 20 | 25 g/1 oz/½ cup | trace | 2 | low | 92 |

| Food | Carbo-hydrate g | Portion size | Fat g | Protein g | Fibre | kCalories per portion |
|---|---|---|---|---|---|---|
| Corn flakes, with semi-skimmed milk | 27 | 5 heaped tbsp | 2 | 6 | low | 149 |
| Corn flakes, with skimmed milk | 27 | 5 heaped tbsp | trace | 6 | low | 133 |
| **Corn flakes cereal and chocolate milk bar** | 18 | 1 bar | 4 | 2 | low | 118 |
| **Corn fritters** | 16 | 1 fritter | 2 | 2 | med | 91 |
| **Corn kernels,** canned, drained *See also* Sweetcorn | 27 | 3 heaped tbsp | 1 | 3 | med | 122 |
| **Corn pops**, dry | 22 | 25 g/1 oz/½ cup | trace | 1 | low | 90 |
| Corn pops, with semi-skimmed milk | 38 | 5 heaped tbsp | 3 | 7 | low | 209 |
| Corn pops, with skimmed milk | 38 | 5 heaped tbsp | 1 | 7 | low | 193 |
| **Corn pops,** chocolate, dry | 20 | 25 g/1 oz/½ cup | 1 | 1 | low | 97 |
| Corn pops, chocolate, with semi-skimmed milk | 38 | 5 heaped tbsp | 4 | 6 | low | 213 |
| Corn pops, chocolate, with skimmed milk | 38 | 5 heaped tbsp | 2 | 6 | low | 197 |
| **Corn puff snacks,** all flavours | 27 | 1 small bag | 16 | 3 | low | 259 (average) |
| **Corn salad** | trace | 1 handful | trace | trace | low | 3 |
| **Cornbread** | 22 | 1 average piece | 5 | 4 | med | 153 |
| **Corned beef** | trace | 1 med slice | 3 | 7 | 0 | 54 |
| **Corned beef hash** | 22 | 1 average serving | 24 | 21 | med | 387 |

| Food | Carbo-hydrate g | Portion size | Fat g | Protein g | Fibre | kCalories per portion |
|------|------|------|------|------|------|------|
| **Cornetto,** all flavours | 26 | 1 cornet | 10 | 3 | low | 198 (average) |
| **Cornflour pudding** | 26 | 1 average serving | 2 | 6 | low | 134 |
| **Cornichons** *See* Gherkins | | | | | | |
| **Cornish crab soup,** canned | 25 | 2 ladlefuls | trace | 6 | low | 118 |
| **Cornish hen** *See* Poussin | | | | | | |
| **Cornish ice cream** | 6 | 1 scoop | 2 | 1 | 0 | 80 |
| **Cornish pasties** | 48 | 1 pasty | 32 | 12 | med | 515 |
| **Cornish wafers** | 5 | 1 wafer | 3 | 1 | low | 47 |
| **Cornmeal** *See* Polenta | | | | | | |
| **Cornmeal muffins** | 23 | 1 muffin | 6 | 4 | low | 154 |
| **Cornmeal pancakes** | 15 | 1 pancake | 3 | 3 | low | 97 |
| **Corn on the cob,** steamed or boiled | 17 | 1 cob | 2 | 4 | med | 99 |
| Corn on the cob, with butter | 17 | 1 cob | 10 | 4 | med | 173 |
| Corn on the cob, with low-fat spread | 17 | 1 cob | 6 | 4 | med | 138 |
| **Coronation chicken** | 15 | 1 average serving | 5 | 40 | low | 266 |
| **Cottage cheese** | 2 | 1 small tub | 4 | 14 | 0 | 98 |
| Cottage cheese, flavoured | 3 | 1 small tub | 4 | 13 | 0 | 95 |
| Cottage cheese, low-fat | 3 | 1 small tub | 1 | 13 | 0 | 78 |
| Cottage cheese, low-fat, flavoured | 3 | 1 small tub | 1 | 12 | 0 | 75 |

| Food | Carbo-hydrate g | Portion size | Fat g | Protein g | Fibre | kCalories per portion |
|---|---|---|---|---|---|---|
| **Cottage loaf** | 15 | 1 med slice | 1 | 3 | low | 74 |
| **Cottage pie** | 25 | 1 average serving | 19 | 24 | med | 330 |
| **Coulibiac** | 30 | 1 average slice | 25 | 12 | low | 380 |
| **Country store**, dry | 17 | 25 g/1 oz/¼ cup | 1 | 2 | med | 87 |
| Country store, with semi-skimmed milk | 33 | 3 heaped tbsp | 4 | 8 | high | 197 |
| Country store, with skimmed milk | 33 | 3 heaped tbsp | 2 | 8 | high | 181 |
| **Courgettes** (zucchini), fried (sautéed) | 3 | 3 heaped tbsp | 5 | 3 | med | 63 |
| Courgettes, steamed or boiled | 2 | 3 heaped tbsp | trace | 2 | med | 19 |
| Courgettes, stuffed | 12 | 2 halves | 8 | 5 | med | 134 |
| Courgettes provençal | 8 | 3 heaped tbsp | 3 | 3 | med | 69 |
| **Couscous** | 29 | 3 heaped tbsp | 4 | 6 | med | 177 |
| **Couscous salad** | 23 | 3 heaped tbsp | 6 | 5 | high | 159 |
| **Crab**, dressed | 17 | 1 med crab | 16 | 63 | low | 459 |
| Crab, dressed, canned | 0 | ½ small can | 3 | 3 | 0 | 21 |
| Crab, white meat | 0 | ½ small can | 1 | 18 | 0 | 81 |
| **Crab and mayonnaise sandwiches** | 34 | 1 round | 29 | 15 | med | 447 |
| **Crab bisque**, home-made | 26 | 2 ladlefuls | 7 | 6 | low | 185 |
| **Crab cakes** | trace | 1 cake | 4 | 12 | 0 | 93 |
| **Crab cocktail** | 7 | 1 average serving | 3 | 10 | med | 102 |
| **Crab sandwiches** | 34 | 1 round | 18 | 14 | med | 344 |

| Food | Carbo-hydrate g | Portion size | Fat g | Protein g | Fibre | kCalories per portion |
|---|---|---|---|---|---|---|
| **Crabapple jelly** (clear conserve) | 13 | 1 level tbsp | trace | trace | 0 | 55 |
| **Crabsticks** | 1 | 1 stick | trace | 2 | 0 | 12 |
| **Cracked wheat** See Bulgar | | | | | | |
| **Crackerbread** | 4 | 1 piece | trace | trace | low | 20 |
| **Crackers,** wholemeal See also Biscuits and individual names, e.g. Ritz | 5 | 1 cracker | 1 | 1 | med | 29 |
| **Cranberries**, dried | 12 | 1 small handful | trace | trace | high | 48 |
| Cranberries, stewed with sugar | 18 | 3 heaped tbsp | trace | trace | low | 70 |
| **Cranberry jelly** (clear conserve) | 10 | 1 level tbsp | 0 | trace | low | 38 |
| **Cranberry juice drink** | 25 | 1 tumbler | 0 | trace | 0 | 104 |
| Cranberry juice drink, light | 11 | 1 tumbler | 0 | trace | 0 | 48 |
| **Cranberry sauce** | 6 | 1 tbsp | 0 | trace | low | 24 |
| **Crayfish**, boiled | 0 | ½ crayfish | 2 | 30 | 0 | 148 |
| **Cream**, aerosol | trace | 1 level tbsp | 5 | trace | 0 | 46 |
| Cream, canned | trace | 1 level tbsp | 4 | trace | 0 | 36 |
| Cream, clotted | trace | 1 level tbsp | 9 | trace | 0 | 88 |
| Cream, double (heavy) | trace | 1 tbsp | 7 | trace | 0 | 67 |
| Cream, half | 1 | 1 tbsp | 2 | trace | 0 | 22 |
| Cream, single (light) | 1 | 1 tbsp | 3 | trace | 0 | 30 |

| Food | Carbo-hydrate g | Portion size | Fat g | Protein g | Fibre | kCalories per portion |
|---|---|---|---|---|---|---|
| Cream, soured (dairy sour) | 1 | 1 level tbsp | 3 | trace | 0 | 31 |
| Cream, sweetened, imitation | 1 | 1 level tbsp | 4 | trace | 0 | 28 |
| Cream, whipping | trace | 1 tbsp | 6 | trace | 0 | 56 |
| Cream cake | 43 | 1 individual cake | 17 | 6 | low | 337 |
| Cream cheese | trace | 1 good spoonful | 12 | 1 | 0 | 110 |
| Cream crackers | 6 | 1 cracker | 1 | 1 | low | 39 |
| Cream crowdie | 14 | 1 serving | 52 | 3 | med | 691 |
| Cream of wheat *See* Semolina | | | | | | |
| Cream soda | 14 | 1 tumbler | trace | trace | low | 58 |
| Cream soups, canned, all flavours *See also individual entries, e.g.* Cream of tomato soup | 9 | 2 ladlefuls | 8 | 2 | low | 110 (average) |
| Crème brûlée | 18 | 1 average serving | 50 | 1 | 0 | 492 |
| Crème caramel | 26 | 1 individual pot | 2 | 4 | 0 | 136 |
| Crème de cassis | 7 | 1 single measure | 0 | trace | 0 | 65 |
| Crème de menthe | 14 | 1 single measure | trace | 0 | 0 | 125 |
| Creme egg, chocolate | 28 | 1 egg | 6 | 2 | 0 | 163 |
| Crème fraîche | trace | 1 level tbsp | 6 | trace | 0 | 56 |
| Crème fraîche, low-fat | 1 | 1 level tbsp | 2 | trace | 0 | 25 |
| Crêpe, plain | 14 | 1 crêpe | 7 | 2 | low | 122 |
| Crêpes suzette | 28 | 2 pancakes | 12 | 4 | med | 317 |
| Crispbread, rye | 6 | 1 cracker | trace | 1 | med | 27 |

| Food | Carbo-hydrate g | Portion size | Fat g | Protein g | Fibre | kCalories per portion |
|------|------|------|------|------|------|------|
| Crispbread, starch-reduced | 3 | 1 cracker | trace | trace | low | 15 |
| Crispbread, wheat | 7 | 1 cracker | trace | 1 | low | 35 |
| **Crispie cakes** | 11 | 1 cake | 3 | 1 | low | 69 |
| **Crisps** (potato chips), all flavours | 12 | 1 small bag | 9 | 1 | med | 136 (average) |
| Crisps, low-fat, all flavours | 16 | 1 small bag | 5 | 2 | med | 114 (average) |
| **Crispy chicken sandwich** | 54 | 1 portion | 27 | 23 | med | 500 |
| **Crispy chicken strips** | 18 | 3 strips | 16 | 26 | low | 300 |
| **Crispy duck with pancakes** | 32 | 1 serving plus 6 pancakes | 42 | 39 | high | 665 |
| **Crispy noodles** | 50 | 1 average serving | 17 | 4 | low | 374 |
| **Crispy vegetable fingers** | 5 | 1 finger | 2 | 1 | low | 45 |
| **Croissant**, all-butter | 20 | 1 croissant | 10 | 4 | low | 185 |
| Croissant, apple | 21 | 1 croissant | 5 | 4 | med | 144 |
| Croissant, chocolate | 26 | 1 croissant | 13 | 4 | low | 236 |
| Croissant, mini | 15 | 1 croissant | 8 | 3 | low | 140 |
| Croissant, raisin | 27 | 1 croissant | 10 | 4 | med | 212 |
| **Croque monsieur** | 36 | 1 round | 27 | 20 | med | 438 |
| **Croquette potatoes**, fried (sautéed) | 22 | 2 croquettes | 13 | 4 | med | 214 |
| Croquette potatoes, frozen, baked | 14 | 2 croquettes | 3 | 2 | low | 90 |
| **Crostini**, garlic | 5 | 1 average slice | 1 | 1 | low | 31 |
| Crostini, mushroom | 16 | 1 average slice | 2 | 3 | low | 92 |

| Food | Carbo-hydrate g | Portion size | Fat g | Protein g | Fibre | kCalories per portion |
|---|---|---|---|---|---|---|
| **Croûtons** | 7 | 1 level tbsp | 5 | 1 | low | 75 |
| **Crown roast of lamb** | 0 | 2 cutlets | 40 | 30 | 0 | 488 |
| **Crudités** | 8 | 1 good handful | 0 | 1 | med | 35 |
| Crudités, with aioli | 8 | 1 average serving | 23 | 1 | med | 272 |
| **Crumpet** | 10 | 1 crumpet | 0 | 3 | low | 80 |
| Crumpet, toasted, with butter | 10 | 1 crumpet | 4 | 3 | low | 117 |
| Crumpet, toasted, with low-fat spread | 10 | 1 crumpet | 2 | 4 | low | 99 |
| **Crunchie** chocolate bar | 30 | 1 standard bar | 8 | 2 | 0 | 195 |
| **Crunchy bran**, dry | 13 | 25 g/1 oz/½ cup | 1 | 3 | high | 74 |
| Crunchy bran, with semi-skimmed milk | 27 | 5 heaped tbsp | 4 | 9 | high | 175 |
| Crunchy bran, with skimmed milk | 27 | 5 heaped tbsp | 2 | 9 | high | 159 |
| **Crunchy cereal bars**, all flavours | 17 | 1 bar | 7 | 2 | med | 146 (average) |
| **Crunchy mixed grain cereal**, with nuts and raisins, dry | 16 | 25 g/1 oz/¼ cup | 3 | 2 | high | 97 |
| Crunchy mixed grain cereal, with nuts and raisins and semi-skimmed milk | 37 | 3 heaped tbsp | 7 | 9 | high | 250 |
| Crunchy mixed grain cereal, with nuts and raisins and skimmed milk | 37 | 3 heaped tbsp | 5 | 9 | high | 234 |

| Food | Carbo-hydrate g | Portion size | Fat g | Protein g | Fibre | kCalories per portion |
|---|---|---|---|---|---|---|
| **Crunchy nut corn flakes**, dry | 20 | 25 g/1 oz/½ cup | 1 | 2 | low | 97 |
| Crunchy nut corn flakes, with semi-skimmed milk | 39 | 5 heaped tbsp | 3 | 7 | low | 213 |
| Crunchy nut corn flakes, with skimmed milk | 39 | 5 heaped tbsp | 1 | 7 | low | 197 |
| **Cucumber** | 1 | 5 med slices | 0 | 0 | low | 4 |
| **Cucumber and yoghurt soup** | 9 | 2 ladlefuls | 3 | 5 | low | 78 |
| **Cucumber sandwiches** | 35 | 1 round | 17 | 5 | med | 308 |
| **Cullen skink** | 16 | 2 ladlefuls | 6 | 13 | low | 170 |
| **Cumberland butter** | 29 | 1 level tbsp | 22 | 0 | 0 | 53 |
| **Cumberland sauce** | 14 | 1 level tbsp | trace | trace | 0 | 64 |
| **Cumberland sausage**, fried (sautéed) | 11 | 1 sausage | 24 | 14 | low | 317 |
| **Cupcakes**, iced (frosted) | 37 | 1 cake | 3 | 1 | low | 179 |
| **Curaçao** | 7 | 1 single measure | 0 | trace | 0 | 78 |
| **Curd cheese** | trace | 1 good spoonful | trace | 4 | 0 | 30 |
| **Curd**, lemon or orange | 9 | 1 level tbsp | 1 | trace | low | 42 |
| **Curly endive** (frisée) | 2 | 1 good handful | trace | trace | med | 6 |
| **Curly kale**, steamed or boiled | 1 | 3 heaped tbsp | 1 | 2 | med | 24 |
| **Curly wurly** chocolate bar | 20 | 1 standard bar | 5 | 1 | 0 | 125 |

| Food | Carbo-hydrate g | Portion size | Fat g | Protein g | Fibre | kCalories per portion |
|------|------|------|------|------|------|------|
| **Currant bread** | 13 | 1 medium slice | 2 | 2 | low | 72 |
| Currant bread, with butter | 13 | 1 medium slice | 10 | 2 | low | 146 |
| Currant bread, with low-fat spread | 13 | 1 medium slice | 6 | 3 | low | 111 |
| **Currant bun** | 26 | 1 bun | 4 | 4 | med | 148 |
| Currant bun, with butter | 26 | 1 bun, 1 small knob | 12 | 4 | med | 222 |
| Currant bun, with low-fat spread | 26 | 1 bun, 1 small knob | 8 | 4 | med | 187 |
| **Currant cake** | 29 | 1 average slice | 6 | 2 | med | 177 |
| **Currants** | 10 | 1 small handful | trace | trace | high | 40 |
| **Curried beans** | 31 | 1 small can | 1 | 10 | high | 168 |
| **Curried chicken and rice salad** | 43 | 1 average serving | 6 | 42 | high | 390 |
| **Curried fruit chutney** | 4 | 1 level tbsp | trace | trace | low | 19 |
| **Curry sauce** | 5 | 5 level tbsp | 4 | 1 | low | 58 |
| **Custard**, canned/ carton | 11 | 5 level tbsp | 2 | 2 | low | 71 |
| Custard, chocolate | 11 | 5 level tbsp | 2 | 2 | low | 71 |
| Custard, egg, baked | 12 | 1 average serving | 7 | 6 | 0 | 130 |
| Custard, made with powder and semi-skimmed milk | 13 | 5 level tbsp | trace | 3 | low | 75 |
| Custard, made with powder and skimmed milk | 13 | 5 level tbsp | 2 | 3 | low | 59 |
| **Custard apple** | 25 | 1 fruit | 1 | 2 | med | 101 |
| **Custard creams** | 8 | 1 biscuit (cookie) | 3 | 1 | low | 57 |

| Food | Carbo-hydrate g | Portion size | Fat g | Protein g | Fibre | kCalories per portion |
|------|------|------|------|------|------|------|
| **Custard sauce**, made with semi-skimmed milk | 7 | 5 level tbsp | 2 | 2 | 0 | 62 |
| Custard sauce, made with skimmed milk | 7 | 5 level tbsp | 1 | 2 | 0 | 52 |
| **Custard tart** | 44 | 1 individual tart | 20 | 8 | med | 373 |
| **Custard-style yoghurt** | 3 | 1 individual pot | 13 | 8 | 0 | 161 |
| **Cuttlefish**, grilled (broiled) | 2 | 1 average serving | 2 | 56 | 0 | 278 |

| Food | Carbo-hydrate g | Portion size | Fat g | Protein g | Fibre | kCalories per portion |
|---|---|---|---|---|---|---|
| **Dab**, fried (sautéed) in breadcrumbs | 16 | 1 medium fish | 23 | 28 | low | 378 |
| Dab, grilled (broiled) | 0 | 1 medium fish | 3 | 35 | 0 | 175 |
| **Daiquiri** | 4 | 1 cocktail | 0 | trace | 0 | 111 |
| **Dairy milk chocolate bar** | 28 | 1 standard bar | 14 | 4 | 0 | 255 |
| **Daktyla bread** | 12 | 1 med slice | 1 | 2 | med | 65 |
| **Damsons** | 1 | 1 fruit | trace | trace | med | 3 |
| Damsons, stewed | 6 | 3 heaped tbsp | trace | 1 | med | 27 |
| Damsons, stewed with sugar | 19 | 3 heaped tbsp | trace | 1 | med | 107 |
| **Damson jam** (conserve) | 10 | 1 level tbsp | 0 | trace | 0 | 39 |
| **Damson pie** | 14 | 1 average slice | 39 | 3 | med | 290 |
| **Dandelion and burdock** | 13 | 1 tumbler | trace | 0 | low | 56 |
| Dandelion and burdock, low-calorie | 0 | 1 tumbler | 0 | 0 | 0 | 3 |
| **Danish apple cake** | 32 | 1 average slice | 10 | 3 | high | 252 |
| **Danish blue cheese** | trace | 1 small wedge | 7 | 5 | 0 | 87 |
| **Danish brown bread** | 10 | 1 med slice | trace | 2 | med | 51 |
| **Danish elbo cheese** | trace | 1 small wedge | 7 | 6 | 0 | 86 |
| **Danish lumpfish roe** | 1 | 1 level tbsp | 3 | 4 | 0 | 40 |
| **Danish pastries**, all types | 51 | 1 pastry | 18 | 6 | med | 374 (average) |
| **Danish toaster bread** | 12 | 1 slice | 1 | 2 | low | 65 |

| Food | Carbo-hydrate g | Portion size | Fat g | Protein g | Fibre | kCalories per portion |
|------|------|------|------|------|------|------|
| Danish toaster bread, toasted, with butter | 12 | 1 slice, 1 small knob | 9 | 2 | low | 129 |
| Danish toaster bread, toasted, with low-fat spread | 12 | 1 slice, 1 small knob | 5 | 2 | low | 94 |
| Danish white bread | 10 | 1 med slice | trace | 2 | low | 50 |
| Date squares | 32 | 1 square | 4 | 4 | high | 170 |
| Dates | 8 | 1 fruit | trace | trace | high | 30 |
| Dates, dried | 10 | 1 fruit | trace | trace | high | 40 |
| Dates, stuffed | 12 | 1 fruit | 4 | 2 | high | 50 |
| Dauphinoise potatoes | 12 | 1 average serving | 15 | 14 | med | 235 |
| Derby cheese | trace | 1 small wedge | 8 | 6 | 0 | 100 |
| Devilled chicken | 6 | 1 average serving | 12 | 48 | 0 | 309 |
| Devilled kidneys | 2 | 1 average serving | 7 | 21 | 0 | 158 |
| Devil's food cake | 40 | 1 average slice | 8 | 3 | low | 255 |
| Devils on horseback | 3 | 1 roll | 4 | 1 | low | 52 |
| Dhal | 21 | 3 heaped tbsp | 6 | 7 | high | 162 |
| Diet coke | 0 | 1 tumbler | 0 | 0 | 0 | 1 |
| Diet pepsi | trace | 1 tumbler | trace | 0 | 1 | 1 |
| Digestive biscuits (graham crackers) | 10 | 1 biscuit (cookie) | 3 | 1 | low | 73 |
| Digestive caramels, chocolate | 11 | 1 biscuit | 4 | 1 | med | 81 |
| Digestive creams | 8 | 1 biscuit (cookie) | 3 | 1 | low | 63 |
| Dijon mustard | trace | 1 level tsp | trace | trace | low | 8 |

| Food | Carbo-hydrate g | Portion size | Fat g | Protein g | Fibre | kCalories per portion |
|---|---|---|---|---|---|---|
| **Dill pickled cucumbers** | 3 | 1 pickle | trace | trace | low | 15 |
| **Dim sum**, assorted | 6 | 1 piece | 2 | 3 | low | 49 (average) |
| **Ditali** (pasta shapes), dried, boiled | 42 | 1 average serving | 1 | 7 | med | 198 |
| Ditali, fresh, boiled | 45 | 1 average serving | 2 | 9 | med | 235 |
| **Dogfish**, fried (sautéed), in batter | 13 | 1 piece of fillet | 33 | 29 | low | 464 |
| **Dolcelatte cheese** | trace | 1 small wedge | 10 | 4 | 0 | 106 |
| **Dolmas** | 19 | 2 rolls | 9 | 18 | high | 221 |
| **Donor kebab**, in pitta bread | 32 | 1 kebab plus 1 bread | 38 | 33 | med | 588 |
| **Dorset blue cheese** | trace | 1 small wedge | 7 | 5 | 0 | 87 |
| **Double chocolate chip muffin** | 48 | 1 muffin | 20 | 5 | low | 397 |
| **Double decker** chocolate bar | 32 | 1 bar | 10 | 3 | 0 | 235 |
| **Double Gloucester cheese** | trace | 1 small wedge | 8 | 6 | 0 | 101 |
| **Doughnut**, apple | 29 | 1 doughnut | 12 | 4 | low | 243 |
| Doughnut, chocolate | 26 | 1 doughnut | 18 | 3 | med | 270 |
| Doughnut, cream | 43 | 1 doughnut | 15 | 4 | low | 265 |
| Doughnut, iced (frosted) | 42 | 1 doughnut | 12 | 4 | low | 286 |
| Doughnut, jam (jelly) | 37 | 1 doughnut | 11 | 4 | low | 252 |
| Doughnut, mini | 7 | 1 doughnut | 3 | 1 | low | 59 |
| Doughnut, plain, ring | 27 | 1 doughnut | 12 | 4 | low | 236 |

| Food | Carbo-hydrate g | Portion size | Fat g | Protein g | Fibre | kCalories per portion |
|------|------|------|------|------|------|------|
| **Dover sole**, fried (sautéed), in seasoned flour | 8 | 1 medium fish | 13 | 25 | low | 342 |
| Dover sole, grilled (broiled) | 0 | 1 medium fish | 9 | 29 | 0 | 202 |
| **Dr Pepper** soft drink | 21 | 1 tumbler | 0 | trace | 0 | 78 |
| Dr Pepper, diet | 0 | 1 tumbler | 0 | 0 | 0 | 1 |
| **Drambuie** | 7 | 1 single measure | 0 | trace | 0 | 85 |
| **Dream topping**, made with semi-skimmed milk | 5 | 3 heaped tbsp | 6 | 2 | low | 75 |
| Dream topping, made with skimmed milk | 5 | 3 heaped tbsp | 4 | 2 | low | 66 |
| Dream topping, sugar-free, made with semi-skimmed milk | 5 | 3 heaped tbsp | 5 | 3 | low | 75 |
| Dream topping, sugar-free, made with skimmed milk | 5 | 3 heaped tbsp | 3 | 3 | 0 | 70 |
| **Dressed crab** | 17 | 1 med crab | 16 | 63 | low | 459 |
| Dressed crab, canned | 0 | ½ small can | 3 | 3 | 0 | 21 |
| **Dried fruit compôte** | 33 | 3 heaped tbsp | trace | 2 | high | 127 |
| **Drifter** chocolate bar | 40 | 1 standard bar | 13 | 3 | low | 292 |
| **Drinking (sweetened) chocolate**, made with semi-skimmed milk | 27 | 1 mug | 5 | 9 | low | 177 |

| Food | Carbo-hydrate g | Portion size | Fat g | Protein g | Fibre | kCalories per portion |
|---|---|---|---|---|---|---|
| Drinking chocolate, made with skimmed milk | 27 | 1 mug | 1 | 9 | low | 146 |
| Drinking chocolate, instant, made with water | 18 | 1 mug | 4 | 3 | low | 119 |
| Drinking yoghurt | 26 | 1 tumbler | trace | 6 | 0 | 124 |
| Drop scone (small pancake) | 6 | 1 pancake | 2 | 1 | low | 44 |
| Dry-cured Belgian ham | 0 | 1 thin slice | 1 | 4 | 0 | 21 |
| Dry-roasted peanuts | 1 | 1 small handful | 7 | 4 | high | 88 |
| Dublin Bay prawns (saltwater crayfish), cooked | 0 | 1 prawn | trace | 2 | 0 | 10 |
| Dubonnet, red | 8 | 1 double measure | 0 | trace | 0 | 75 |
| Duchesse potatoes | 17 | 2 pieces | 5 | 5 | med | 165 |
| Duck, breast, grilled (broiled), without skin | 0 | 1 medium breast | 19 | 50 | 0 | 378 |
| Duck, breast, grilled, with skin | 0 | 1 medium breast | 58 | 37 | 0 | 678 |
| Duck, crispy Peking | 32 | 1 serving plus 6 pancakes | 42 | 39 | high | 665 |
| Duck, roast, with skin | 0 | 1/4 duck | 65 | 44 | 0 | 763 |
| Duck à l'orange | 8 | 1/4 duck | 69 | 49 | med | 856 |
| Duck eggs, boiled | trace | 1 egg | 8 | 9 | 0 | 106 |
| Duck liver pâté | 1 | 1 average serving | 14 | 6 | 0 | 158 |
| Duck soup, home-made | 7 | 2 ladlefuls | 4 | 12 | 0 | 114 |

| Food | Carbo-hydrate g | Portion size | Fat g | Protein g | Fibre | kCalories per portion |
|------|-----------------|--------------|-------|-----------|-------|-----------------------|
| **Duck with cherries** | 4 | ¼ duck | 65 | 44 | low | 836 |
| **Dumplings** | 9 | 1 dumpling | 1 | 1 | low | 73 |
| **Dundee cake** | 58 | 1 average slice | 17 | 6 | med | 397 |
| **Dunlop cheese** | trace | 1 small wedge | 9 | 6 | 0 | 103 |
| **Dutch apple tart** | 34 | 1 average slice | 10 | 3 | med | 237 |

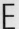 

| Food | Carbo-hydrate g | Portion size | Fat g | Protein g | Fibre | kCalories per portion |
|---|---|---|---|---|---|---|
| **Easter biscuits** (cookies) | 16 | 1 biscuit | 4 | 1 | low | 58 |
| **Eccles cake** | 26 | 1 cake | 12 | 2 | med | 214 |
| **Echo** chocolate bar | 15 | 1 standard bar | 7 | 2 | low | 132 |
| **Eclair**, chocolate | 18 | 1 éclair | 21 | 4 | low | 277 |
| **Edam (Dutch) cheese** | trace | 1 small wedge | 6 | 6 | 0 | 83 |
| **Eel pie mash**, with pea gravy | 35 | 1 average serving | 25 | 17 | med | 434 |
| **Eels**, jellied | trace | 1 small serving | 6 | 6 | 0 | 70 |
| Eels, silver, stewed | 0 | 1 average serving | 13 | 25 | 0 | 320 |
| Eels, smoked | 0 | 1 average serving | 13 | 10 | 0 | 167 |
| **Egg**, baked, with cream | trace | 1 egg | 13 | 7 | 0 | 151 |
| Egg, boiled | trace | 1 egg | 6 | 7 | 0 | 84 |
| Egg, coddled | trace | 1 egg | 6 | 7 | 0 | 84 |
| Egg, curried | 5 | 2 eggs | 16 | 15 | low | 226 |
| Egg, fried (sautéed) | trace | 1 egg | 8 | 8 | 0 | 102 |
| Egg, pickled | trace | 1 egg | 6 | 7 | 0 | 84 |
| Egg, poached | trace | 1 egg | 6 | 7 | 0 | 84 |
| Egg, scotch | 16 | 1 egg | 20 | 14 | low | 301 |
| Egg, scrambled | 1 | 2 eggs | 28 | 13 | 0 | 308 |
| Egg, stuffed | trace | 2 halves | 17 | 7 | 0 | 187 |
| Egg and cress sandwiches | 68 | 1 round | 23 | 13 | med | 392 |
| **Egg custard tart** | 44 | 1 individual tart | 20 | 8 | med | 373 |
| **Egg custard**, baked | 12 | 1 average serving | 7 | 6 | 0 | 130 |

| Food | Carbo-hydrate g | Portion size | Fat g | Protein g | Fibre | kCalories per portion |
|---|---|---|---|---|---|---|
| Egg custard, packet, made up with semi-skimmed milk | 23 | 1 average serving | 6 | 5 | 0 | 168 |
| Egg custard, packet, made up with skimmed milk | 23 | 1 average serving | 4 | 5 | 0 | 149 |
| Egg fried rice | 46 | 1 average serving | 19 | 7 | low | 374 |
| Egg mayonnaise | trace | 1 egg | 29 | 7 | 0 | 290 |
| Egg mayonnaise sandwiches | 34 | 1 round | 34 | 13 | med | 491 |
| Egg mcmuffin | 27 | 1 portion | 12 | 17 | med | 290 |
| Egg nog | 7 | 1 single measure | 2 | 1 | 0 | 68 |
| Egg noodles, chinese | 26 | 1 average serving | 1 | 4 | med | 124 |
| Egg salad | 5 | 2 eggs | 12 | 16 | high | 200 |
| Egg salad, dressed | 5 | 2 eggs | 29 | 16 | high | 297 |
| Egg sauce | 8 | 5 level tbsp | 7 | 5 | low | 117 |
| Eggplant See Aubergine | | | | | | |
| Eggs benedict | 43 | 1 egg | 17 | 22 | med | 402 |
| Eggs florentine | 7 | 1 egg | 16 | 16 | med | 239 |
| Eggy bread | 17 | 1 medium slice | 18 | 6 | low | 213 |
| Elderflower pressé | 12 | 1 wine glass | trace | trace | 0 | 50 |
| Elmlea cream blend, double (heavy) | trace | 1 tbsp | 6 | trace | low | 61 |
| Elmlea, single (light) | trace | 1 tbsp | 5 | trace | low | 48 |
| Elmlea, whipping | trace | 1 tbsp | 4 | trace | low | 43 |
| Elmlea light, double (heavy) | 1 | 1 tbsp | 4 | trace | low | 37 |

| Food | Carbo-hydrate g | Portion size | Fat g | Protein g | Fibre | kCalories per portion |
|------|------|------|------|------|------|------|
| Elmlea light, single (light) | trace | 1 tbsp | 3 | trace | low | 17 |
| Elmlea light, whipping | trace | 1 tbsp | 2 | trace | low | 28 |
| **Emmental (Swiss) cheese** | 1 | 1 small wedge | 8 | 7 | 0 | 105 |
| **Enchiladas** *See individual fillings, e.g.* Cheese enchiladas | | | | | | |
| **English muffin** | 27 | 1 muffin | 1 | 5 | med | 127 |
| English muffin, toasted, with butter | 27 | 1 muffin | 9 | 5 | med | 200 |
| English muffin, toasted, with low-fat spread | 27 | 1 muffin | 5 | 6 | med | `166 |
| **English mustard** | trace | 1 level tsp | trace | trace | low | 7 |
| **Escargots à la bourguignonne** | trace | 6 snails | 25 | 12 | low | 311 |
| **Escarole** | 2 | 1 good handful | trace | trace | med | 6 |
| **Esrom cheese** | trace | 1 small wedge | 7 | 5 | 0 | 84 |
| **Evaporated milk** | 151 | 100 ml/3½ fl oz/ scant ½ cup | 8 | 8 | 9 | 0 |
| Evaporated milk, light | 80 | 100 ml/3½ fl oz/ scant ½ cup | 10 | 11 | trace | 0 |
| **Everton mints** | 4 | 1 mint | trace | trace | 0 | 21 |
| **Everton toffee** | 1 | 1 toffee | 0 | trace | 0 | 20 |
| **Eve's pudding** | 40 | 1 average serving | 6 | 3 | med | 222 |
| **Exotic fruit drink** | 22 | 1 tumbler | trace | trace | 0 | 90 |

| Food | Carbo-hydrate g | Portion size | Fat g | Protein g | Fibre | kCalories per portion |
|------|-----------------|--------------|-------|-----------|-------|-----------------------|
| **Fab** ice lolly | 17 | 1 lolly | 3 | 1 | 0 | 99 |
| **Faggots** | 23 | 2 faggots | 27 | 16 | low | 402 |
| **Fairy cakes** | 22 | 1 individual cake | 2 | 2 | low | 105 |
| **Fajitas** *See individual fillings, e.g.* Beef fajitas | | | | | | |
| **Falafels** | 11 | 2 falafels | 9 | 5 | high | 140 |
| **Fanta** orange | 22 | 1 tumbler | 0 | 0 | 0 | 85 |
| Fanta orange, diet | 0 | 1 tumbler | 0 | 0 | 0 | 6 |
| **Farfalle** (pasta shapes), dried, boiled | 42 | 1 average serving | 1 | 7 | med | 198 |
| Farfalle, fresh, boiled | 45 | 1 average serving | 2 | 9 | med | 235 |
| **Farmhouse loaf** | 15 | 1 medium slice | 1 | 3 | low | 74 |
| **Farmhouse vegetable soup**, canned | 16 | 2 ladlefuls | 1 | 4 | med | **90** |
| Farmhouse vegetable soup, packet | 25 | 2 ladlefuls | 1 | 4 | high | 119 |
| **Feast** ice lolly | 23 | 1 lolly | 13 | 3 | low | 313 |
| **Fennel** | 4 | 1 head | 3 | 2 | med | 27 |
| Fennel, au gratin | 8 | 1 average serving | 10 | 7 | med | 145 |
| Fennel, steamed or boiled | 1 | ½ head | trace | 1 | med | 11 |
| **Feta cheese** | trace | 1 small chunk | 5 | 4 | 0 | 62 |
| Feta cheese, with olives | trace | 1 piece of each | 2 | 1 | low | 19 |

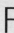
| Food | Carbo- hydrate g | Portion size | Fat g | Protein g | Fibre | kCalories per portion |
|---|---|---|---|---|---|---|
| **Fettuccine** (pasta ribbons), dried, boiled | 51 | 1 average serving | 2 | 8 | med | 239 |
| Fettuccine, fresh, boiled | 57 | 1 average serving | 2 | 11 | med | 301 |
| **Fibre 1**, dry | 13 | 25 g/1 oz/½ cup | 1 | 3 | high | 66 |
| Fibre 1, with semi- skimmed milk | 26 | 5 heaped tbsp | 3 | 9 | high | 166 |
| Fibre 1, with skimmed milk | 26 | 5 heaped tbsp | 1 | 9 | high | 150 |
| **Fig roll biscuit** (cookie) | 11 | 1 roll | 2 | 1 | med | 61 |
| **Figgy duff** | 80 | 1 average serving | 28 | 9 | high | 581 |
| **Figs** | 5 | 1 fig | trace | 1 | high | 24 |
| Figs, canned in syrup | 25 | 3 heaped tbsp | trace | trace | high | 88 |
| Figs, dried, ready- to-eat | 11 | 1 fig | trace | 1 | high | 45 |
| Figs, dried, stewed | 29 | 3 heaped tbsp | 1 | 3 | high | 103 |
| Figs, dried, stewed with sugar | 34 | 3 heaped tbsp | 1 | 3 | high | 143 |
| Figs, with parma ham | 11 | 1 fig plus 2 slices of ham | 2 | 9 | high | 87 |
| **Filberts** See Hazelnuts | | | | | | |
| **Filet-o-fish** | 41 | 1 portion | 18 | 17 | med | 389 |
| **Fillet steak** See Steak, fillet | | | | | | |
| **Fingers**, milk chocolate | 6 | 1 biscuit (cookie) | 1 | trace | low | 38 |
| **Finger rolls** | 21 | 1 roll | 2 | 4 | low | 107 |

| Food | Carbo-hydrate g | Portion size | Fat g | Protein g | Fibre | kCalories per portion |
|---|---|---|---|---|---|---|
| **Finnan haddie** | 0 | 1 fish | 1 | 34 | 0 | 148 |
| Fish and chips, deep-fried, chip-shop-style | 68 | 1 average serving | 46 | 54 | high | 891 |
| **Fish cakes, salmon**, fried (sautéed) | 15 | 1 cake | 11 | 8 | low | 213 |
| Fish cakes, salmon, grilled (broiled) | 17 | 1 cake | 7 | 10 | low | 192 |
| Fish cakes, white fish, fried | 15 | 1 cake | 10 | 9 | low | 188 |
| Fish cakes, white fish, grilled | 17 | 1 cake | 6 | 11 | low | 169 |
| **Fish chowder** | 60 | 2 ladlefuls | 10 | 44 | med | 285 |
| **Fish fingers**, fried (sautéed) | 3 | 1 finger | 3 | 3 | low | 47 |
| Fish fingers, grilled (broiled) | 4 | 1 finger | 2 | 3 | low | 43 |
| **Fish goujons** | 6 | 6 goujons | 14 | 37 | low | 304 |
| **Fish kebabs** | 0 | 1 kebab | 1 | 21 | 0 | 95 |
| **Fish mornay** | 13 | 1 average serving | 21 | 11 | low | 239 |
| **Fish mousse** | 6 | 1 average serving | 15 | 10 | low | 180 |
| **Fish paste** | trace | 1 level tbsp | 1 | 2 | low | 25 |
| **Fish pie**, topped with pastry (paste) | 27 | 1 average serving | 25 | 14 | low | 384 |
| Fish pie, topped with potato | 37 | 1 average serving | 9 | 24 | med | 315 |
| **Fish soup** | 21 | 2 ladlefuls | 2 | 16 | med | 159 |
| **Fish stew** | 43 | 1 average serving | 5 | 30 | med | 330 |
| **Fish sticks** | 7 | 1 stick | 3 | 4 | 0 | 76 |

| Food | Carbo-hydrate g | Portion size | Fat g | Protein g | Fibre | kCalories per portion |
|---|---|---|---|---|---|---|
| **Flageolet beans**, canned, drained | 21 | 3 heaped tbsp | 1 | 7 | high | 98 |
| Flageolet beans, dried, soaked and cooked | 23 | 3 heaped tbsp | 1 | 8 | high | 104 |
| **Flake** chocolate bar | 19 | 1 standard bar | 10 | 3 | 0 | 180 |
| **Flan**, fruit, any flavour | 40 | 1 average slice | 6 | 3 | low | 222 |
| **Flapjack** | 48 | 1 piece | 23 | 6 | high | 417 |
| **Florida cocktail** | 10 | 1 average serving | trace | trace | low | 56 |
| **Flounder**, fried (sautéed), in breadcrumbs | 16 | 1 small fish | 23 | 28 | low | 378 |
| Flounder, grilled (broiled) | 0 | 1 small fish | 2 | 35 | 0 | 175 |
| **Focaccia** bread | 30 | 1 medium slice | 1 | 3 | med | 139 |
| **Fois gras** | 1 | 1 average serving | 14 | 6 | 0 | 158 |
| **Fondant creams** | 7 | 1 sweet (candy) | 0 | trace | 0 | 25 |
| **Fondant icing** (frosting) | 25 | 25 g/1 oz | 0 | 0 | 0 | 100 |
| **Fondue**, cheese | 8 | 1 average serving | 29 | 30 | 0 | 492 |
| Fondue, cheese, with French bread | 62 | 1 average serving plus 10 cubes of bread | 31 | 40 | med | 762 |
| **Fontina cheese** | trace | 1 small wedge | 9 | 7 | 0 | 110 |
| **Forcemeat balls** | 10 | 2 balls | 7 | 3 | low | 115 |
| **Four cheese pizza** | 36 | 1 large slice | 17 | 13 | med | 334 |
| **Four cheese pasta sauce** | 76 | ¼ jar | 13 | 17 | med | 500 |
| **Four seasons pizza** | 32 | 1 large slice | 16 | 12 | med | 342 |

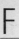

| Food | Carbo-hydrate g | Portion size | Fat g | Protein g | Fibre | kCalories per portion |
|---|---|---|---|---|---|---|
| **Frankfurter** | 2 | 1 frankfurter | 15 | 9 | low | 186 |
| Frankfurter, canned | 1 | 1 frankfurter | 7 | 3 | low | 82 |
| **French (green) beans**, canned, drained | 4 | 3 heaped tbsp | trace | 1 | med | 22 |
| French beans, steamed or boiled | 5 | 3 heaped tbsp | trace | 2 | high | 25 |
| **French dressing** | 0 | 1 tbsp | 17 | trace | 0 | 97 |
| French dressing, low-calorie | 1 | 1 tbsp | trace | trace | 0 | 5 |
| **French fancies**, fondant-iced (frosted) | 25 | 1 cake | 5 | 1 | low | 150 |
| **French fries**, thin, from burger outlets *See also* Chips | 28 | 1 average serving | 9 | 3 | med | 206 |
| **French mustard** | 1 | 1 level tsp | trace | trace | low | 7 |
| **French onion soup**, canned | 11 | 2 ladlefuls | trace | 2 | low | 48 |
| French onion soup, home-made | 8 | 2 ladlefuls | 6 | 2 | low | 94 |
| French onion soup, packet | 20 | 2 ladlefuls | 1 | 2 | low | 104 |
| French onion soup, with cheese croûtes | 21 | 2 ladlefuls plus 1 croûte | 8 | 9 | low | 226 |
| **French stick** | 27 | 1 thick slice | 1 | 5 | low | 135 |
| **French toast** | 17 | 1 medium slice | 18 | 6 | low | 213 |
| **Fried (sautéed) bread** | 17 | 1 medium slice | 11 | 3 | low | 181 |

| Food | Carbo-hydrate g | Portion size | Fat g | Protein g | Fibre | kCalories per portion |
|---|---|---|---|---|---|---|
| **Fried (sautéed) egg sandwiches** | 34 | 1 round | 25 | 13 | med | 406 |
| **Fried rice** *See* Rice, Egg fried rice *and* Special fried rice | | | | | | |
| **Fries** *See* Chips | | | | | | |
| **Frisée** *See* Curly endive | | | | | | |
| **Frito misto** | 43 | 1 average serving | 11 | 24 | low | 338 |
| **Frittata** | 17 | 2 eggs | 22 | 16 | med | 328 |
| **Frogs' legs**, fried (sautéed) | 0 | 2 legs | 10 | 22 | low | 178 |
| **Fromage blanc** | trace | 1 good spoonful | trace | 2 | 0 | 24 |
| **Fromage frais** | 6 | 1 individual pot | 7 | 7 | 0 | 113 |
| Fromage frais, flavoured | 14 | 1 individual pot | 6 | 7 | low | 131 |
| Fromage frais, low-fat | 7 | 1 individual pot | trace | 8 | low | 58 |
| Fromage frais, low-fat, flavoured | 7 | 1 individual pot | trace | 8 | low | 58 |
| **Frosted shreddies**, dry | 20 | 25 g/1 oz/½ cup | trace | 2 | high | 91 |
| Frosted shreddies, with semi-skimmed milk | 43 | 5 heaped tbsp | 3 | 7 | high | 224 |
| Frosted shreddies, with skimmed milk | 43 | 5 heaped tbsp | 1 | 7 | high | 208 |
| **Frosted wheats**, dry | 17 | 25 g/1 oz/½ cup | trace | 2 | high | 80 |
| Frosted wheats, with semi-skimmed milk | 34 | 5 heaped tbsp | 3 | 8 | high | 185 |

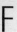 

| Food | Carbo-hydrate g | Portion size | Fat g | Protein g | Fibre | kCalories per portion |
|---|---|---|---|---|---|---|
| Frosted wheats, with skimmed milk | 34 | 5 heaped tbsp | 1 | 8 | high | 169 |
| **Frosties**, dry | 22 | 25 g/1 oz/½ cup | trace | 1 | low | 95 |
| Frosties, with semi-skimmed milk | 41 | 5 heaped tbsp | 2 | 6 | low | 209 |
| Frosties, with skimmed milk | 41 | 5 heaped tbsp | trace | 6 | low | 193 |
| **Frosties cereal and milk bar** | 18 | 1 bar | 4 | 3 | low | 121 |
| **Frosting** See Icing | | | | | | |
| **Fruit cake**, light | 58 | 1 average slice | 13 | 5 | med | 354 |
| Fruit cake, rich *See also* Christmas cake | 60 | 1 average slice | 11 | 4 | med | 341 |
| **Fruit chewy sweets** (candies) | 38 | 1 tube | 4 | trace | 0 | 185 |
| **Fruit cobbler** | 46 | 1 average serving | 7 | 4 | med | 255 |
| **Fruit cocktail,** canned in natural juice | 15 | 3 heaped tbsp | trace | trace | low | 57 |
| Fruit cocktail, canned in syrup | 20 | 3 heaped tbsp | trace | trace | low | 77 |
| **Fruit corner** yoghurt dessert | 26 | 1 indv carton | 7 | 6 | low | 219 |
| **Fruit flan**, made with pastry (paste) | 24 | 1 average slice | 6 | 2 | low | 153 |
| Fruit flan, made with sponge | 40 | 1 average slice | 1 | 3 | low | 222 |
| **Fruit gums** | 32 | 1 tube | 0 | 2 | 0 | 134 |
| **Fruit 'n' fibre**, dry | 17 | 25 g/1 oz/½ cup | 1 | 2 | high | 87 |

| Food | Carbo-hydrate g | Portion size | Fat g | Protein g | Fibre | kCalories per portion |
|---|---|---|---|---|---|---|
| Fruit 'n' fibre, with semi-skimmed milk | 34 | 5 heaped tbsp | 4 | 8 | high | 197 |
| Fruit 'n' fibre, with skimmed milk | 34 | 5 heaped tbsp | 2 | 8 | high | 181 |
| **Fruit pastilles** | 35 | 1 tube | 0 | 2 | 0 | 147 |
| **Fruit pie** | 39 | 1 individual pie | 8 | 2 | med | 241 |
| **Fruit punch** | 15 | 1 wine glass | 0 | 0 | low | 59 |
| **Fruit salad**, canned in natural juice | 7 | 3 heaped tbsp | trace | trace | low | 29 |
| Fruit salad, canned in syrup | 15 | 3 heaped tbsp | trace | trace | low | 57 |
| Fruit salad, dried | 40 | 3 heaped tbsp | trace | 3 | high | 145 |
| Fruit salad, dried, stewed | 26 | 3 heaped tbsp | trace | 1 | high | 83 |
| Fruit salad, dried, stewed with sugar | 29 | 3 heaped tbsp | trace | 1 | high | 94 |
| Fruit salad, fresh, in pure juice | 7 | 3 heaped tbsp | trace | 1 | med | 27 |
| Fruit salad, fresh, in syrup | 14 | 3 heaped tbsp | trace | 1 | med | 55 |
| Fruit salad, tropical | 9 | 3 heaped tbsp | 0 | 1 | med | 47 |
| **Fruit scone** (biscuit) | 26 | 1 scone | 5 | 4 | med | 158 |
| Fruit scone, with butter | 26 | 1 scone | 13 | 4 | med | 232 |
| Fruit scone, with low-fat spread | 26 | 1 scone | 9 | 5 | med | 197 |
| **Fruit shortcake** | 7 | 1 biscuit (cookie) | 2 | 1 | low | 52 |

| Food | Carbo-hydrate g | Portion size | Fat g | Protein g | Fibre | kCalories per portion |
|------|------|------|------|------|------|------|
| **Fruit squash** *See individual flavours, e.g.* Orange squash | | | | | | |
| **Fruitful shredded wheat**, dry | 17 | 25 g/1 oz/½ cup | 1 | 2 | high | 88 |
| Fruitful shredded wheat, with semi-skimmed milk | 34 | 3 heaped tbsp | 4 | 8 | high | 202 |
| Fruitful shredded wheat, with skimmed milk | 34 | 3 heaped tbsp | 2 | 8 | high | 186 |
| **Fruitibix**, dry | 18 | 25 g/1 oz/½ cup | 1 | 2 | high | 88 |
| Fruitibix, with semi-skimmed milk | 34 | 3 heaped tbsp | 3 | 8 | high | 200 |
| Fruitibix, with skimmed milk | 34 | 3 heaped tbsp | 1 | 8 | high | 184 |
| **Fudge** *See also individual flavours, e.g.* Chocolate fudge | 14 | 1 square | 2 | trace | 0 | 77 |
| **Fudge brownie** | 62 | 1 brownie | 20 | 5 | low | 394 |
| **Ful medames beans**, dried, soaked and cooked | 20 | 3 heaped tbsp | 1 | 9 | high | 116 |
| **Fusilli** (pasta spirals), dried, boiled | 51 | 1 average serving | 2 | 8 | med | 239 |
| Fusilli, fresh, boiled | 57 | 1 average serving | 2 | 11 | med | 301 |

| Food | Carbo-hydrate g | Portion size | Fat g | Protein g | Fibre | kCalories per portion |
|---|---|---|---|---|---|---|
| **Gaelic coffee** | 7 | 1 wine glass | 14 | 1 | 0 | 218 |
| **Gala pie** | 37 | 1 average slice | 68 | 15 | med | 564 |
| **Galaxy** chocolate bar, all flavours | 27 | 1 standard bar | 14 | 4 | 0 | 250 (average) |
| **Galaxy cake bar** | 20 | 1 cake bar | 10 | 2 | low | 178 |
| Galaxy cake bar, caramel | 20 | 1 cake bar | 7 | 2 | low | 148 |
| **Galaxy double nut and raisin bar** | 26 | 1 standard bar | 14 | 4 | 0 | 246 |
| **Galaxy ice cream** | 28 | 1 ice cream bar | 19 | 4 | 0 | 302 |
| **Galaxy muffin** | 42 | 1 muffin | 18 | 5 | low | 356 |
| **Game chips** | 25 | 10 chips | 19 | 3 | med | 273 |
| **Game pie** | 49 | 1 average serving | 35 | 21 | med | 606 |
| **Game soup**, canned | 10 | 2 ladlefuls | 4 | 5 | low | 88 |
| **Gammon**, honey-roast | 4 | 2 thick slices | 6 | 25 | 0 | 174 |
| Gammon, lean, boiled | 0 | 2 thick slices | 5 | 29 | 0 | 167 |
| Gammon, rasher (slice), fried (sautéed) | 0 | 1 rasher | 9 | 22 | 0 | 171 |
| Gammon, rasher, grilled (broiled) | 0 | 1 rasher | 8 | 22 | 0 | 141 |
| Gammon, steak, grilled | 0 | 1 med steak | 9 | 54 | 0 | 301 |
| **Gammon with pineapple** | 6 | 1 med steak plus 1 pineapple slice | 9 | 54 | 0 | 324 |
| **Gammon and egg** | trace | 1 med steak plus 1 egg | 17 | 62 | 0 | 403 |

| Food | Carbo-hydrate g | Portion size | Fat g | Protein g | Fibre | kCalories per portion |
|------|------|------|------|------|------|------|
| **Garbanzos** *See* Chick peas | | | | | | |
| **Garibaldi biscuits** (cookies) | 7 | 1 biscuit | 1 | trace | low | 41 |
| **Garlic** | 1 | 1 clove | trace | trace | low | 5 |
| **Garlic and herb soft cheese** | 1 | 1 good spoonful | 7 | 2 | low | 77 |
| **Garlic bread** | 7 | 1 small slice | 4 | 1 | low | 73 |
| **Garlic butter** | trace | 1 level tbsp | 12 | trace | low | 112 |
| **Garlic chicken** | 3 | 1 breast | 16 | 40 | low | 316 |
| **Garlic mayonnaise** | trace | 2 level tbsp | 23 | trace | 0 | 237 |
| **Garlic sausage** | trace | 1 med slice | 1 | 1 | low | 12 |
| **Gazpacho** | trace | 2 ladlefuls | 7 | 3 | med | 136 |
| **Genoa cake** | 56 | 1 average slice | 16 | 5 | med | 383 |
| **German smoked cheese** | trace | 1 small wedge | 3 | 4 | 0 | 60 |
| **Ghee** | trace | 25 g/1 oz/2 tbsp | 25 | trace | 0 | 224 |
| **Gherkins** (cornichons) | 1 | 1 gherkin | trace | trace | low | 4 |
| **Gin** | trace | 1 single measure | 0 | trace | 0 | 55 |
| **Gin and dry martini** | 3 | 1 cocktail | trace | trace | 0 | 114 |
| **Gin and lime** | 15 | 1 single measure | 0 | trace | 0 | 111 |
| **Gin and orange** | 7 | 1 single measure | 0 | trace | 0 | 108 |
| Gin and sweet martini | 8 | 1 cocktail | 0 | trace | 0 | 75 |
| Gin and tonic | 5 | 1 single measure plus 1 mixer | 0 | trace | 0 | 76 |
| Gin and tonic, low-calorie | trace | 1 single measure plus 1 mixer | trace | trace | 0 | 56 |

| Food | Carbo-hydrate g | Portion size | Fat g | Protein g | Fibre | kCalories per portion |
|---|---|---|---|---|---|---|
| **Ginger**, chocolate | 7 | 1 piece | trace | trace | low | 30 |
| Ginger, crystallised | 4 | 1 piece | 0 | trace | low | 30 |
| Ginger, stem, in syrup | 2 | 1 piece | trace | trace | low | 30 |
| **Ginger ale,** american | 10 | 1 tumbler | 0 | 0 | 0 | 44 |
| Ginger ale, dry | 8 | 1 tumbler | 0 | 0 | 0 | 32 |
| Ginger ale, low-calorie | trace | 1 tumbler | trace | trace | 0 | 1 |
| **Ginger beer** | 24 | 1 tumbler | 0 | 0 | 0 | 98 |
| **Ginger cake** | 60 | 1 average slice | 15 | 3 | med | 388 |
| **Ginger cake bar** | 22 | 1 cake bar | 4 | 1 | low | 128 |
| **Ginger ice cream** | 11 | 1 scoop | 4 | 2 | low | 89 |
| **Ginger nuts** | 9 | 1 biscuit (cookie) | 2 | 1 | low | 56 |
| Ginger nuts, milk or plain (semi-sweet) chocolate | 10 | 1 biscuit | 3 | 1 | low | 70 |
| **Ginger snaps** | 6 | 1 biscuit (cookie) | 1 | trace | low | 37 |
| **Ginger wine** | 16 | 1 double measure | 0 | trace | 0 | 200 |
| **Gingerbread** | 28 | 1 average slice | 7 | 2 | low | 180 |
| **Gingerbread men** | 34 | 1 man | 11 | 4 | low | 249 |
| **Gipsy creams** | 8 | 1 biscuit (cookie) | 3 | 1 | low | 64 |
| **Gjetost cheese** | 12 | 1 small wedge | 8 | 3 | 0 | 132 |
| **Glacé (candied) cherries** | 4 | 1 cherry | trace | trace | low | 13 |
| **Glacé (candied) fruits** | 4 | 1 piece | trace | trace | low | 13 |
| **Glacé icing** (frosting) | 14 | 1 level tbsp | 0 | 0 | 0 | 56 |

| Food | Carbo-hydrate g | Portion size | Fat g | Protein g | Fibre | kCalories per portion |
|------|------|------|------|------|------|------|
| **Globe artichoke**, whole, steamed or boiled *See also* Artichokes | 3 | 1 med artichoke | 0 | 0 | med | 70 |
| Globe artichoke heart, canned, drained | 1 | 1 heart | trace | 1 | med | 8 |
| **Glucose**, powdered or liquid | 13 | 1 level tbsp | 0 | trace | 0 | 48 |
| **Gnocchi** | 13 | 1 average serving | 12 | 3 | low | 213 |
| Gnocchi, with butter and Parmesan | 13 | 1 average serving | 29 | 9 | low | 385 |
| **Goats' cheese**, hard | 1 | 1 small wedge | 10 | 9 | 0 | 128 |
| Goats' cheese, soft | trace | 1 good spoonful | 12 | 10 | 0 | 152 |
| **Goats' milk** | 12 | 300 ml/½ pt/ 1¼ cups | 10 | 9 | 0 | 180 |
| **Golden cutlets** (smoked whiting), poached | 0 | 1 med fillet | 1 | 21 | 0 | 166 |
| **Golden grahams**, dry | 20 | 25 g/1 oz/½ cup | 1 | 1 | low | 93 |
| Golden grahams, with semi-skimmed milk | 30 | 5 heaped tbsp | 3 | 6 | low | 172 |
| Golden grahams, with skimmed milk | 30 | 5 heaped tbsp | 1 | 6 | low | 156 |
| **Golden nuggets**, dry | 22 | 25 g/1 oz/½ cup | trace | 1 | low | 95 |
| Golden nuggets, with semi-skimmed milk | 32 | 5 heaped tbsp | 2 | 6 | low | 174 |

| Food | Carbo-hydrate g | Portion size | Fat g | Protein g | Fibre | kCalories per portion |
|---|---|---|---|---|---|---|
| Golden nuggets, with skimmed milk | 32 | 5 heaped tbsp | trace | 6 | low | 158 |
| **Golden raisins** *See* Sultanas | | | | | | |
| **Golden (light corn) syrup** | 12 | 1 level tbsp | 0 | trace | 0 | 45 |
| **Golden syrup cake bar** | 60 | 1 cake bar | 14 | 4 | med | 385 |
| Golden syrup cake bar, mini | 22 | 1 cake bar | 4 | 1 | low | 126 |
| **Goose**, roast, without skin | 0 | 3 med slices | 22 | 29 | 0 | 319 |
| **Gooseberries** | 3 | 3 heaped tbsp | trace | 1 | med | 19 |
| Gooseberries, canned in syrup | 18 | 3 heaped tbsp | trace | trace | med | 73 |
| Gooseberries, stewed | 2 | 3 heaped tbsp | trace | 1 | med | 16 |
| Gooseberries, stewed with sugar | 13 | 3 heaped tbsp | trace | 1 | med | 54 |
| **Gooseberry fool** | 20 | 1 average serving | 9 | 3 | med | 183 |
| **Gooseberry pie** | 40 | 1 average slice | 16 | 4 | med | 314 |
| **Gooseberry sauce** | trace | 1 level tbsp | 4 | trace | med | 42 |
| **Gorgonzola cheese** | trace | 1 small wedge | 10 | 4 | 0 | 106 |
| **Gouda cheese** | trace | 1 small wedge | 8 | 6 | 0 | 94 |
| **Gougère**, cheese | 8 | 1 average serving | 24 | 16 | low | 239 |
| **Goulash, Hungarian** | 16 | 1 average serving | 22 | 28 | med | 406 |
| **Graham crackers** *See* Digestive biscuits | | | | | | |
| **Grainy mustard** | 1 | 1 level tsp | trace | 2 | low | 7 |

| Food | Carbo-hydrate g | Portion size | Fat g | Protein g | Fibre | kCalories per portion |
|---|---|---|---|---|---|---|
| **Granary bread** | 18 | 1 medium slice | 1 | 4 | med | 94 |
| **Grand Marnier** | 7 | 1 single measure | 0 | trace | 0 | 78 |
| **Granda padano cheese** | trace | 1 small wedge | 8 | 10 | 0 | 113 |
| **Granola**, dry | 17 | 25 g/1 oz/¼ cup | 1 | 3 | high | 89 |
| Granola, with semi-skimmed milk | 40 | 3 heaped tbsp | 5 | 10 | high | 236 |
| Granola, with skimmed milk | 40 | 3 heaped tbsp | 3 | 10 | high | 226 |
| **Grape juice** | 23 | 1 tumbler | trace | 1 | 0 | 92 |
| Grape juice, red | 23 | 1 tumbler | trace | 1 | 0 | 92 |
| Grape juice, red, sparkling | 16 | 1 wine glass | 0 | trace | 0 | 61 |
| Grape juice, white | 23 | 1 tumbler | trace | 1 | 0 | 92 |
| Grape juice, white, sparkling | 16 | 1 wine glass | 0 | trace | 0 | 61 |
| **Grapefruit** | 12 | 1 fruit | trace | 2 | med | 48 |
| Grapefruit, canned in natural juice | 7 | 3 heaped tbsp | trace | 1 | low | 30 |
| Grapefruit, canned in syrup | 15 | 3 heaped tbsp | trace | trace | low | 60 |
| Grapefruit, with port | 8 | ½ grapefruit | trace | 1 | med | 47 |
| Grapefruit, with sugar | 16 | ½ grapefruit | trace | 1 | med | 64 |
| Grapefruit, with sugar, grilled (broiled) | 16 | ½ grapefruit | trace | 1 | med | 64 |
| **Grapefruit cocktail** | 18 | 1 average serving | trace | trace | low | 72 |
| **Grapefruit drink**, sparkling | 24 | 1 tumbler | 0 | 0 | 0 | 88 |

| Food | Carbo-hydrate g | Portion size | Fat g | Protein g | Fibre | kCalories per portion |
|---|---|---|---|---|---|---|
| **Grapefruit juice** | 17 | 1 tumbler | trace | 1 | low | 66 |
| **Grapefruit juice drink** | 18 | 1 tumbler | trace | trace | low | 72 |
| **Grapenuts**, dry | 20 | 25 g/1 oz/½ cup | trace | 2 | med | 86 |
| Grapenuts, with semi-skimmed milk | 26 | 3 heaped tbsp | 2 | 8 | med | 195 |
| Grapenuts, with skimmed milk | 26 | 3 heaped tbsp | trace | 8 | med | 183 |
| **Grapes**, black | 15 | 1 small bunch | trace | trace | low | 60 |
| Grapes, green | 15 | 1 small bunch | trace | trace | low | 60 |
| **Grappa** | 6 | 1 single measure | 0 | trace | 0 | 79 |
| **Gravlax** | 4 | 1 average serving | 21 | 34 | 0 | 336 |
| **Gravy**, made with giblets or meat juices | 2 | 5 tbsp | 4 | 4 | low | 56 |
| Gravy, made with granules | 2 | 5 tbsp | 2 | trace | low | 25 |
| Gravy, thin | trace | 5 tbsp | trace | trace | 0 | 2 |
| **Greek pastries** | 40 | 1 piece | 17 | 5 | med | 322 |
| **Greek slow-roasted lamb** *See* Kleftiko | | | | | | |
| **Greek pork stew** *See* Afelia | | | | | | |
| **Greek village salad** | 5 | 1 average serving | 8 | 6 | high | 108 |
| **Greek-style yoghurt**, cows' | 5 | 1 individual pot | 13 | 8 | 0 | 161 |
| Greek-style yoghurt, sheep's | 8 | 1 individual pot | 10 | 6 | 0 | 149 |

| Food | Carbo-hydrate g | Portion size | Fat g | Protein g | Fibre | kCalories per portion |
|------|------|------|------|------|------|------|
| Greek-style yoghurt, with honey | 15 | 1 individual pot | 9 | 6 | 0 | 158 |
| **Green beans** *See* French (green) beans | | | | | | |
| **Green chartreuse** | 7 | 1 single measure | 0 | trace | 0 | 78 |
| **Green salad** | 2 | 1 average serving | trace | 1 | med | 14 |
| Green salad, dressed | 2 | 1 average serving | 17 | 1 | med | 111 |
| **Greengage** | 2 | 1 fruit | trace | trace | med | 13 |
| **Greengage pie** | 39 | 1 average slice | 14 | 3 | med | 290 |
| **Greengages,** canned in natural juice | 11 | 3 heaped tbsp | trace | trace | med | 51 |
| Greengages, canned in syrup | 16 | 3 heaped tbsp | trace | trace | med | 69 |
| Greengages, stewed | 6 | 3 heaped tbsp | trace | 1 | med | 37 |
| Greengages, stewed with sugar | 19 | 3 heaped tbsp | trace | 1 | med | 117 |
| **Grenadine syrup,** undiluted | 9 | 1 tbsp | 0 | trace | 0 | 35 |
| **Griddle scones** (biscuits) | 6 | 1 scone | 2 | 1 | low | 44 |
| **Grillsteak,** minced (ground) beef, grilled (broiled) | 8 | 1 steak | 12 | 11 | low | 185 |
| Grillsteak, minced lamb, grilled (broiled) | 1 | 1 steak | 13 | 14 | 0 | 175 |
| **Ground beef** *See* Beef, minced | | | | | | |

| Food | Carbo-hydrate g | Portion size | Fat g | Protein g | Fibre | kCalories per portion |
|------|-----------------|--------------|-------|-----------|-------|-----------------------|
| **Ground rice pudding**, made with semi-skimmed milk | **40** | 1 average serving | 11 | 8 | low | 205 |
| Ground rice pudding, made with skimmed milk | **40** | 1 average serving | trace | 8 | low | 186 |
| **Grouper**, grilled (broiled) | **6** | 1 piece of fillet | 3 | 50 | 0 | 238 |
| **Grouse**, roast | **0** | 1 small bird | 14 | 82 | 0 | 456 |
| **Gruyère (Swiss) cheese** | **trace** | 1 small wedge | 9 | 8 | 0 | 117 |
| **Guacamole** | **1** | 1 average serving | 45 | 1 | med | 408 |
| **Guard of honour**, stuffed | **10** | 2 lamb cutlets | 42 | 30 | low | 550 |
| **Guava** | **5** | 1 medium fruit | trace | 1 | high | 26 |
| Guava, canned in natural juice | **11** | 3 heaped tbsp | 0 | trace | high | 48 |
| Guava, canned in syrup | **16** | 3 heaped tbsp | 0 | trace | high | 60 |
| **Guinea fowl**, roast | 0 | ¼ bird | 14 | 74 | 0 | 480 |
| **Guinness** | 6 | 1 small | trace | 1 | 0 | 117 |

| Food | Carbo-hydrate g | Portion size | Fat g | Protein g | Fibre | kCalories per portion |
|---|---|---|---|---|---|---|
| **Haddock**, fried (sautéed), in batter | 19 | 1 piece of fillet | 26 | 46 | low | 490 |
| Haddock, fried, in breadcrumbs | 9 | 1 piece of fillet | 26 | 53 | low | 435 |
| Haddock, poached or steamed | 0 | 1 piece of fillet | 1 | 40 | 0 | 171 |
| Haddock, smoked, poached | 0 | 1 piece of fillet | 1 | 41 | 0 | 176 |
| **Haggis** | 19 | 1 average serving | 22 | 11 | low | 310 |
| **Hake**, fried (sautéed), in batter | 19 | 1 piece of fillet | 26 | 49 | 0 | 497 |
| Hake, poached or steamed | 0 | 1 piece of fillet | 7 | 42 | 0 | 164 |
| **Halibut**, grilled (broiled) | 0 | 1 piece of fillet | 7 | 42 | 0 | 231 |
| Halibut, poached or steamed | 0 | 1 piece of fillet | 7 | 42 | 0 | 229 |
| **Halloumi cheese** | 1 | 1 thick slice | 7 | 7 | 0 | 98 |
| Halva | 23 | ¼ block | 16 | 7 | low | 265 |
| **Ham**, boiled | 0 | 2 thick slices | 5 | 29 | 0 | 167 |
| Ham, canned | 0 | 1 medium slice | 2 | 9 | 0 | 60 |
| Ham, ready-sliced, no added water | trace | 1 medium slice | 1 | 6 | 0 | 37 |
| Ham, honey-roast | 4 | 2 thick slices | 6 | 25 | low | 174 |
| **Ham and cheese quiche** | 24 | 1 large slice | 32 | 23 | low | 476 |
| **Ham and chopped pork loaf** | trace | 1 medium slice | 3 | 2 | low | 35 |
| **Ham and mushroom pizza**, deep-pan | 35 | 1 large slice | 11 | 8 | med | 292 |

| Food | Carbo-hydrate g | Portion size | Fat g | Protein g | Fibre | kCalories per portion |
|---|---|---|---|---|---|---|
| Ham and mushroom pizza, thin-crust | 26 | 1 large slice | 9 | 8 | med | 242 |
| **Ham and pineapple pizza**, deep-pan | 31 | 1 large slice | 11 | 8 | med | 276 |
| Ham and pineapple pizza, thin-crust | 22 | 1 large slice | 9 | 8 | med | 226 |
| **Ham and tomato quiche** | 25 | 1 large slice | 32 | 23 | low | 479 |
| **Ham sandwiches** | 34 | 1 round | 18 | 11 | med | 341 |
| **Hamburger**, retail | 33 | 1 burger in a bun | 8 | 13 | med | 253 |
| Hamburger, home-made | 25 | 1 burger in a bun | 14 | 31 | low | 437 |
| **Hare**, jugged | 7 | 1 average serving | 30 | 30 | low | 420 |
| Hare, roast | 0 | 1 average serving | 9 | 30 | 0 | 193 |
| Hare, stewed | 0 | 1 average serving | 8 | 30 | 0 | 192 |
| **Haricot (navy) beans**, canned, drained | 17 | 3 heaped tbsp | trace | 7 | high | 92 |
| Haricot beans, dried, soaked and cooked | 17 | 3 heaped tbsp | trace | 7 | high | 95 |
| **Haricot mutton/ lamb** | 24 | 1 average serving | 9 | 21 | med | 252 |
| **Harusami noodles** | 57 | 1 average serving | trace | 2 | low | 251 |
| **Hash browns** | 16 | 1 portion | 8 | 1 | med | 138 |
| **Haslet** | 2 | 1 med slice | 2 | 2 | low | 30 |
| Havarti cheese | 0 | 1 med slice | 9 | 6 | 0 | 100 |
| **Hawaiian pizza**, deep-pan | 31 | 1 large slice | 11 | 8 | med | 276 |
| Hawaiian pizza, thin-crust | 22 | 1 large slice | 9 | 8 | med | 226 |

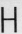

| Food | Carbo-hydrate g | Portion size | Fat g | Protein g | Fibre | kCalories per portion |
|---|---|---|---|---|---|---|
| **Hazelnut (filbert) ice cream** | 12 | 1 scoop | 4 | 2 | low | 91 |
| **Hazelnuts**, shelled | 1 | 25 g/1 oz/¼ cup | 16 | 3 | high | 162 |
| **Hearts**, braised | 8 | 1 average serving | 8 | 33 | high | 190 |
| Hearts, roast, stuffed | 4 | 1 average serving | 19 | 27 | low | 295 |
| Hearts, stewed | 0 | 1 average serving | 6 | 31 | 0 | 179 |
| **Herring**, grilled (broiled) | 0 | 1 medium fish | 13 | 21 | 0 | 202 |
| Herring, filleted, fried (sautéed), in oatmeal | 2 | 1 medium fish | 22 | 34 | low | 351 |
| Herring, pickled | 1 | 1 small fillet | 3 | 2 | 0 | 39 |
| Herring, rollmop | 6 | 1 roll | 12 | 12 | 0 | 180 |
| Herring, soused | 6 | 1 roll | 12 | 12 | 0 | 180 |
| **Herring roes**, fried (sautéed) | 5 | 1 average serving | 16 | 21 | low | 244 |
| Herring roes, on buttered toast | 23 | 1 average serving +1 slice of toast | 25 | 24 | low | 399 |
| **Hobnobs** | 9 | 1 biscuit (cookie) | 3 | 1 | low | 69 |
| Hobnobs, chocolate | 12 | 1 biscuit | 5 | 1 | low | 96 |
| Hobnob creams, chocolate or vanilla | 8 | 1 biscuit | 3 | 1 | low | 63 |
| **Hoisin sauce** | 6 | 1 level tbsp | trace | trace | low | 27 |
| Hollandaise sauce | trace | 3 level tbsp | 25 | 8 | 0 | 214 |
| **Homewheat biscuits** (cookies), chocolate | 11 | 1 biscuit | 4 | 1 | low | 87 |
| Homewheat biscuits, chocolate, mini | 2 | 1 biscuit | 1 | trace | low | 18 |

| Food | Carbo-hydrate g | Portion size | Fat g | Protein g | Fibre | kCalories per portion |
|---|---|---|---|---|---|---|
| **Honey** | 13 | 1 level tbsp | 0 | trace | 0 | 43 |
| **Honey cake** | 14 | 1 slice | 0 | trace | low | 89 |
| **Honey crispix**, dry | 21 | 25 g/1 oz/½ cup | trace | 1 | low | 95 |
| Honey crispix, with semi-skimmed milk | 33 | 5 heaped tbsp | 3 | 6 | low | 209 |
| Honey crispix, with skimmed milk | 33 | 5 heaped tbsp | 1 | 6 | low | 193 |
| **Honey loops**, dry | 19 | 25 g/1 oz/½ cup | 1 | 2 | med | 92 |
| Honey loops, with semi-skimmed milk | 37 | 5 heaped tbsp | 3 | 7 | med | 205 |
| Honey loops, with skimmed milk | 37 | 5 heaped tbsp | 1 | 7 | med | 189 |
| **Honey mustard** | trace | 1 level tsp | trace | trace | 0 | 7 |
| **Honey nut cheerios**, dry | 20 | 25 g/1 oz/½ cup | 1 | 2 | med | 93 |
| Honey nut cheerios, with semi-skimmed milk | 30 | 5 heaped tbsp | 3 | 6 | med | 172 |
| Honey nut cheerios, with skimmed milk | 30 | 5 heaped tbsp | 1 | 6 | med | 156 |
| **Honey nut corn flakes**, dry | 20 | 25 g/1 oz/½ cup | 1 | 2 | low | 97 |
| Honey nut corn flakes, with semi-skimmed milk | 39 | 5 heaped tbsp | 3 | 7 | low | 213 |
| Honey nut corn flakes, with skimmed milk | 39 | 5 heaped tbsp | 1 | 7 | low | 197 |
| **Honey nut shredded wheat**, dry | 17 | 25 g/1 oz/½ cup | 2 | 3 | high | 95 |

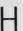 

| Food | Carbo-hydrate g | Portion size | Fat g | Protein g | Fibre | kCalories per portion |
|---|---|---|---|---|---|---|
| **Honey nut shredded wheat**, with semi-skimmed milk | 34 | 3 heaped tbsp | 5 | 8 | high | 210 |
| Honey nut shredded wheat, with skimmed milk | 34 | 3 heaped tbsp | 3 | 8 | high | 194 |
| **Honey rice krispies**, dry | 22 | 25 g/1 oz/½ cup | trace | 1 | low | 35 |
| Honey rice krispies, with semi-skimmed milk | 42 | 5 heaped tbsp | 2 | 6 | low | 209 |
| Honey rice krispies, with skimmed milk | 42 | 5 heaped tbsp | trace | 6 | low | 193 |
| **Honeycomb** | 11 | 1 level tbsp | 1 | trace | 0 | 42 |
| **Honeydew melon** | 15 | 1 large wedge | trace | 1 | med | 63 |
| **Horlicks**, made with semi-skimmed milk | 32 | 1 mug | 5 | 11 | low | 202 |
| Horlicks, made with skimmed milk | 32 | 1 mug | 1 | 11 | low | 170 |
| Horlicks, instant, chocolate, made with water | 21 | 1 mug | 3 | 5 | med | 128 |
| Horlicks, instant, chocolate malted, made with water | 24 | 1 mug | 2 | 3 | med | 129 |
| Horlicks, instant, low-fat, made with water | 25 | 1 mug | 1 | 6 | low | 127 |
| **Horn of plenty mushrooms**, fried (sautéed) | **trace** | 2 good tbsp | 8 | 1 | low | 78 |

| Food | Carbo-hydrate g | Portion size | Fat g | Protein g | Fibre | kCalories per portion |
|---|---|---|---|---|---|---|
| Horn of plenty mushrooms, stewed | trace | 2 good tbsp | trace | 1 | low | 6 |
| **Horseradish**, cream | 1 | 1 level tsp | 1 | trace | low | 11 |
| Horseradish, fresh, grated | 1 | 1 level tbsp | 1 | trace | low | 24 |
| Horseradish, relish | trace | 1 level tsp | trace | trace | low | 5 |
| Horseradish, sauce | 1 | 1 level tsp | trace | trace | low | 8 |
| **Hot and sour soup** | 8 | 2 ladlefuls | 6 | 12 | low | 129 |
| **Hot chocolate** *See* Drinking (sweetened) chocolate | | | | | | |
| **Hot cross bun** | 26 | 1 bun | 4 | 4 | med | 148 |
| Hot cross bun, with butter | 26 | 1 bun | 12 | 4 | med | 222 |
| Hot cross bun, with low-fat spread | 26 | 1 bun | 8 | 4 | med | 187 |
| **Hot dog** | 22 | 1 sausage plus 1 bun | 9 | 7 | med | 189 |
| Hot dog, sausage only | 1 | 1 sausage | 7 | 3 | low | 82 |
| Hot dog, with onions | 4 | 1 sausage plus 1 bun | 10 | 4 | med | 230 |
| **Hot fudge sundae** | 30 | 1 sundae | 5 | 3 | 0 | 180 |
| **Hummus** | 13 | 2 level tbsp | 22 | 10 | high | 280 |
| **Hula hoops** *See* Potato hoops | | | | | | |
| **Hungarian goulash** | 16 | 1 average serving | 22 | 28 | med | 406 |
| **Huss** *See* Rock salmon | | | | | | |

| Food | Carbo-hydrate g | Portion size | Fat g | Protein g | Fibre | kCalories per portion |
|---|---|---|---|---|---|---|
| **Ice cream**, dairy, flavoured | 11 | 1 scoop | 4 | 2 | low | 89 |
| Ice cream, dairy, vanilla | 12 | 1 scoop | 5 | 2 | low | 97 |
| Ice cream, low-calorie, flavoured | 8 | 1 scoop | 3 | 2 | low | 67 |
| Ice cream, low-calorie, vanilla | 9 | 1 scoop | 3 | 1 | low | 71 |
| Ice cream, mixed, multi-flavours | 12 | 1 scoop | 4 | 2 | low | 91 |
| Ice cream, non-dairy, flavoured | 11 | 1 scoop | 4 | 1 | low | 83 |
| Ice cream, non-dairy, vanilla | 11 | 1 scoop | 4 | 2 | low | 89 |
| **Ice cream 99**, with flake bar | 31 | 1 cornet | 13 | 5 | low | 175 |
| **Ice cream bombe** | 18 | 1 average serving | 17 | 4 | 0 | 283 |
| **Ice cream cone**, double | 34 | 2 scoops | 8 | 5 | low | 222 |
| Ice cream cone, single | 22 | 1 scoop | 4 | 3 | low | 131 |
| **Ice cream gâteau** | 23 | 1 average slice | 14 | 3 | low | 227 |
| **Ice lolly**, any flavour | 7 | 1 lolly | trace | trace | 0 | 28 |
| **Ice pop**, large | 17 | 1 lolly | 0 | 0 | 0 | 63 |
| Ice pop, small | 11 | 1 lolly | 0 | 0 | 0 | 42 |
| Ice split, any flavour | 13 | 1 lolly | 3 | 1 | 0 | 83 (average) |
| **Iceberg lettuce** | 1 | 1 good handful | 0 | trace | low | 2 |
| **Iced coffee** | 10 | 1 tumbler | 8 | 6 | 0 | 133 |

| Food | Carbo-hydrate g | Portion size | Fat g | Protein g | Fibre | kCalories per portion |
|---|---|---|---|---|---|---|
| Iced coffee, with sugar | 15 | 1 tumbler | 8 | 6 | 0 | 173 |
| **Iced (frosted) fancies** | 25 | 1 cake | 5 | 1 | low | 150 |
| **Iced gems** | 25 | 1 small bag | 1 | 2 | low | 117 |
| **Iced tea**, with sugar | 20 | 1 tumbler | 0 | 0 | 0 | 89 |
| **Icing** (frosting) *See individual types, e.g.* Fondant icing | | | | | | |
| **Instant whipped dessert**, made with semi-skimmed milk | 14 | 1 average serving | 6 | 3 | low | 103 |
| Instant whipped dessert, made with skimmed milk | 14 | 1 average serving | 3 | 3 | low | 88 |
| Instant whipped dessert, sugar-free, made with semi-skimmed milk | 11 | 1 average serving | 7 | 3 | 0 | 103 |
| Instant whipped dessert, sugar-free, made with skimmed milk | 11 | 1 average serving | 6 | 3 | 0 | 88 |
| **Irish coffee** | 7 | 1 wine glass | 14 | 1 | 0 | 218 |
| **Irish cream liqueur** | 6 | 1 single measure | 5 | 1 | 0 | 102 |
| **Irish stew** | 25 | 1 average serving | 21 | 14 | med | 336 |
| **Irn-bru** | 21 | 1 tumbler | trace | 0 | low | 65 |
| Irn-bru, diet | 2 | 1 tumbler | trace | 0 | low | 8 |
| **Isotonic drink** | 21 | 1 can/carton | 0 | trace | 0 | 92 |
| **Italian pork sausage** | 1 | 1 sausage | 17 | 13 | 0 | 216 |

| Food | Carbo-hydrate g | Portion size | Fat g | Protein g | Fibre | kCalories per portion |
|---|---|---|---|---|---|---|
| **Jacket potato** See also Potato, baked | 64 | 1 large potato | trace | 8 | high | 272 |
| **Jaffa cake** | 9 | 1 individual cake | 1 | 1 | low | 48 |
| Jaffa cake, mini | 5 | 1 small cake | 1 | trace | low | 26 |
| Jaffa cake muffin | 57 | 1 bar | 19 | 4 | low | 416 |
| **Jalousie**, jam (conserve) | 33 | 1 average slice | 20 | 3 | low | 319 |
| Jalousie, mincemeat | 33 | 1 average slice | 21 | 4 | med | 321 |
| **Jam** (conserve), any flavour | 10 | 1 level tbsp | 0 | trace | 0 | 39 |
| Jam, any flavour, reduced-sugar | 5 | 1 level tbsp | trace | trace | 0 | 18 |
| **Jam (jelly) roll**, steamed or baked | 52 | 1 average slice | 19 | 5 | med | 391 |
| **Jam ring biscuits** (cookies) | 9 | 1 biscuit | 2 | 1 | low | 60 |
| **Jam sandwich cake** | 64 | 1 average slice | 5 | 4 | low | 302 |
| **Jam sandwich creams** | 9 | 1 biscuit (cookie) | 3 | 1 | low | 74 |
| **Jam sponge cake** | 64 | 1 average slice | 5 | 4 | low | 302 |
| **Jam tart** | 20 | 1 individual tart | 5 | 1 | low | 130 |
| **Jambalaya** | 61 | 1 average serving | 6 | 41 | high | 468 |
| **Japanese miso soup** | 8 | 2 ladlefuls | 4 | 5 | med | 78 |
| **Jarlsberg cheese** | 1 | 1 small wedge | 8 | 7 | 0 | 105 |
| **Jellied consommé** | 2 | 2 ladlefuls | trace | 5 | 0 | 32 |
| **Jellied eels** | trace | 1 small serving | 6 | 6 | 0 | 70 |
| **Jello** See Jelly | | | | | | |

| Food | Carbo-hydrate g | Portion size | Fat g | Protein g | Fibre | kCalories per portion |
|------|------|------|------|------|------|------|
| **Jelly** (jello), any flavour | 22 | 1 average serving | 0 | 2 | 0 | 91 |
| Jelly, milk, made with semi-skimmed milk | 28 | 1 average serving | 2 | 6 | 0 | 148 |
| Jelly, milk, made with skimmed milk | 28 | 1 average serving | trace | 6 | 0 | 132 |
| Jelly, sugar-free, made up | trace | 1 average serving | trace | 1 | 0 | 8 |
| Jelly, yoghurt | 12 | 1 average serving | 1 | 5 | 0 | 60 |
| **Jelly babies** | 3 | 1 sweet (candy) | 0 | trace | 0 | 15 |
| **Jelly beans** | 3 | 1 bean | 0 | trace | 0 | 11 |
| **Jelly roll** *See* Jam roll *and* Swiss roll | | | | | | |
| **Jelly tots** | 37 | 1 small packet | 0 | trace | 0 | 147 |
| **Jerk chicken** | 15 | 1 average serving | 8 | 32 | high | 256 |
| **Jerusalem artichokes**, steamed or boiled | 11 | 3 heaped tbsp | 0 | 2 | high | 41 |
| **Jugged hare** | 7 | 1 average serving | 30 | 30 | low | 420 |
| **Jumbo shrimp** *See* King prawn | | | | | | |
| **Junket**, made with semi-skimmed milk | 16 | 1 average serving | 4 | 4 | 0 | 120 |
| Junket, made with skimmed milk | 16 | 1 average serving | 2 | 4 | 0 | 101 |
| **Just right**, dry | 19 | 25 g/1 oz/½ cup | 1 | 2 | med | 90 |
| Just right, with semi-skimmed milk | 37 | 5 heaped tbsp | 3 | 7 | med | 201 |
| Just right, with skimmed milk | 37 | 5 heaped tbsp | 1 | 7 | med | 185 |

| Food | Carbo-hydrate g | Portion size | Fat g | Protein g | Fibre | kCalories per portion |
|---|---|---|---|---|---|---|
| **Kalamares**, fried (sautéed), in batter | 19 | 1 average serving | 12 | 14 | low | 235 |
| **Kale**, steamed or boiled | 1 | 3 heaped tbsp | 1 | 2 | med | 24 |
| **Kateifi** | 40 | 1 pastry | 17 | 5 | med | 322 |
| **Kedgeree**, made with smoked fish | 31 | 1 average serving | 24 | 43 | low | 498 |
| Kedgeree, made with white fish | 31 | 1 average serving | 24 | 44 | low | 495 |
| **Kelp** | 1 | 2 good tbsp | trace | trace | low | 4 |
| **Kentucky fried chicken** | 10 | 2 pieces | 27 | 29 | low | 390 |
| **Ketchup** (catsup) | 4 | 1 level tbsp | trace | trace | low | 15 |
| **Kettle chips**, all flavours | 12 | 1 good handful | 9 | 1 | med | 136 (average) |
| **Kidney beans** *See* Red kidney beans | | | | | | |
| **Kidneys**, devilled | 2 | 1 average serving | 7 | 21 | 0 | 158 |
| Kidneys, lambs', fried (sautéed) | 0 | 2 kidneys | 6 | 25 | 0 | 155 |
| Kidneys, lambs', grilled (broiled) | 0 | 2 kidneys | 4 | 26 | 0 | 109 |
| Kidneys, ox, stewed | 0 | 1 average serving | 8 | 26 | 0 | 172 |
| Kidneys, pigs', fried (sautéed) | 0 | 1 kidney | 6 | 25 | 0 | 155 |
| Kidneys, pigs', stewed | 0 | 1 kidney | 6 | 24 | 0 | 153 |
| **Kidneys turbigo** | 2 | 1 average serving | 54 | 48 | low | 363 |
| **Kielbasa sausage**, grilled (broiled) | 1 | 1 med slice | 7 | 3 | 0 | 81 |
| **King cone** | 29 | 1 cone | 7 | 2 | low | 186 |

| Food | Carbo-hydrate g | Portion size | Fat g | Protein g | Fibre | kCalories per portion |
|---|---|---|---|---|---|---|
| **King prawn** (jumbo shrimp) | 0 | 1 prawn | trace | 2 | 0 | 10 |
| King prawn, battered | 3 | 1 prawn | 2 | 2 | low | 45 |
| King prawn, in garlic butter | trace | 1 prawn | 2 | 2 | low | 48 |
| **King prawn masala** | 5 | 1 average serving | 6 | 24 | low | 164 |
| **Kipper**, grilled (broiled) | 0 | 1 medium fish | 9 | 21 | 0 | 166 |
| Kipper, poached or jugged | 0 | 1 medium fish | 9 | 21 | 0 | 166 |
| **Kipper fillets**, boil-in-the-bag | 0 | 1 fillet | 15 | 16 | 0 | 201 |
| Kipper fillets, canned in oil, drained | trace | 1 fillet | 12 | 11 | 0 | 140 |
| **Kipper pâté** | trace | 1 average serving | 17 | 8 | 0 | 190 |
| **Kir** | 8 | 1 wine glass | 0 | trace | 0 | 131 |
| **Kirsch** | trace | 1 single measure | 0 | trace | 0 | 50 |
| **Kit kat chocolate bar** | 13 | 2 fingers | 5 | 1 | low | 107 |
| Kit kat chocolate bar, chunky | 33 | 1 bar | 15 | 4 | low | 282 |
| Kiwi fruit | 11 | 1 fruit | trace | 1 | med | 46 |
| **Kleftiko** (Greek slow-roast lamb with potatoes) | 11 | 1 average serving | 49 | 67 | med | 741 |
| **Knackwurst/ knockwurst** | 1 | 1 sausage | 19 | 8 | 0 | 209 |
| **Knickerbocker glory** | 41 | 1 tall glass | 10 | 8 | low | 273 |
| **Kohlrabi**, steamed or boiled | 5 | 3 heaped tbsp | 0 | 1 | med | 36 |

| Food | Carbo-hydrate g | Portion size | Fat g | Protein g | Fibre | kCalories per portion |
|------|------|------|------|------|------|------|
| **Krackawheat** | 5 | 1 cracker | 2 | 1 | low | 38 |
| **Krispen**, all flavours | 3 | 1 cracker | trace | trace | low | 15 (average) |
| **Kulfi ice cream** | 9 | 1 average serving | 32 | 4 | low | 340 |
| **Kumquat** | 3 | 1 fruit | 0 | 0 | low | 12 |

| Food | Carbo-hydrate g | Portion size | Fat g | Protein g | Fibre | kCalories per portion |
|------|------|------|------|------|------|------|
| **Ladies' fingers** See Okra | | | | | | |
| **Lady fingers** See Boudoir | | | | | | |
| **Lager** | 3 | 1 small | 0 | 1 | 0 | 87 |
| Lager, high-strength | 7 | 1 small | 0 | 1 | 0 | 226 |
| Lager, low-alcohol | 4 | 1 small | 0 | trace | 0 | 70 |
| **Lamb**, breast, roast | 0 | 2 thick slices | 37 | 19 | 0 | 410 |
| Lamb, chop, lean, fried (sautéed) | 0 | 1 chop | 25 | 18 | 0 | 277 |
| Lamb, chop, lean, grilled (broiled) | 0 | 1 chop | 23 | 18 | 0 | 250 |
| Lamb, crown roast | 0 | 2 cutlets | 40 | 30 | 0 | 488 |
| Lamb, cutlet, lean, fried | 0 | 1 cutlet | 22 | 15 | 0 | 267 |
| Lamb, cutlet, lean, grilled | 0 | 1 cutlet | 20 | 15 | 0 | 244 |
| Lamb, grillsteak, grilled | 1 | 1 steak | 13 | 14 | 0 | 175 |
| Lamb, guard of honour | 10 | 2 cutlets | 42 | 30 | low | 550 |
| Lamb, leg, roast, lean and fat | 0 | 2 thick slices | 18 | 26 | 0 | 266 |
| Lamb, leg, roast, lean only | 0 | 2 thick slices | 8 | 29 | 0 | 191 |
| Lamb, minced (ground), stewed | 0 | 1 average serving | 22 | 39 | 0 | 354 |
| Lamb, noisettes, fried | 0 | 2 noisettes | 14 | 28 | 0 | 245 |
| Lamb, noisettes, grilled | 0 | 2 noisettes | 12 | 28 | 0 | 222 |

| Food | Carbo-hydrate g | Portion size | Fat g | Protein g | Fibre | kCalories per portion |
|------|------|------|------|------|------|------|
| Lamb, shank, slow-roasted | 0 | 1 shank | 31 | 45 | 0 | 465 |
| Lamb, shoulder, roast, lean and fat | 0 | 3 medium slices | 26 | 20 | 0 | 316 |
| Lamb, shoulder, roast, lean only | 0 | 3 medium slices | 11 | 24 | 0 | 196 |
| Lamb, steak, fried (sautéed) | 0 | 1 steak | 16 | 51 | 0 | 357 |
| Lamb, steak, grilled (broiled) | 0 | 1 steak | 14 | 51 | 0 | 334 |
| Lamb biryani | 75 | 1 average serving | 51 | 22 | med | 828 |
| Lamb curry | 10 | 1 average serving | 82 | 37 | med | 935 |
| Lamb curry, with rice | 66 | 1 average serving | 84 | 42 | med | 1183 |
| Lamb goulash | 16 | 1 average serving | 26 | 28 | med | 446 |
| Lamb kheema | 5 | 1 average serving | 58 | 29 | low | 656 |
| Lamb rogan josh | 17 | 1 average serving | 41 | 51 | med | 691 |
| Lamb stew | 30 | 1 average serving | 13 | 16 | med | 369 |
| Lamb tagine | 14 | 1 average serving | 54 | 47 | med | 724 |
| Lambrusco | 2 | 1 wine glass | 0 | trace | 0 | 70 |
| Lamingtons | 36 | 1 individual cake | 2 | 3 | med | 233 |
| Lancashire cheese | trace | 1 small wedge | 8 | 58 | 0 | 93 |
| Lancashire hot-pot | 30 | 1 average serving | 13 | 28 | high | 342 |
| Langoustines | 0 | 1 langoustine | trace | 2 | 0 | 10 |
| Langues de chat | 3 | 1 biscuit (cookie) | 1 | trace | low | 28 |
| Lasagne, meat, home-made | 32 | 1 average serving | 44 | 36 | med | 650 |
| Lasagne, meat, ready-prepared | 38 | 1 average serving | 11 | 15 | low | 306 |
| Lasagne, seafood | 32 | 1 average serving | 16 | 22 | high | 351 |

| Food | Carbo-hydrate g | Portion size | Fat g | Protein g | Fibre | kCalories per portion |
|---|---|---|---|---|---|---|
| Lasagne, vegetable | 50 | 1 average serving | 10 | 15 | high | 424 |
| Lassi | 26 | 1 tumbler | trace | 6 | low | 124 |
| Leek | 6 | 1 medium leek | 1 | 4 | high | 44 |
| Leek, roast | 3 | 1 medium leek | 3 | 1 | high | 67 |
| Leek, sliced, steamed or boiled | 3 | 3 heaped tbsp | 1 | 1 | med | 21 |
| Leek and potato soup, canned | 8 | 2 ladlefuls | 6 | 2 | low | 94 |
| Leek and potato soup, home-made | 15 | 2 ladlefuls | 5 | 5 | med | 117 |
| Leek and potato soup, packet | 24 | 2 ladlefuls | 7 | 2 | low | 80 |
| Leek vinaigrette | 3 | 4 small leeks | 23 | 1 | med | 223 |
| Leerdammer cheese | trace | 1 small wedge | 8 | 7 | 0 | 93 |
| Lemon | 2 | 1 fruit | trace | trace | 0 | 12 |
| Lemon and lime, sparkling | 19 | 1 tumbler | trace | trace | 0 | 78 |
| Lemon and lime, sparkling, low-calorie | 2 | 1 tumbler | trace | trace | 0 | 9 |
| Lemon barley water, diluted | 9 | 1 tumbler | trace | trace | 0 | 40 |
| Lemon cake | 54 | 1 average slice | 18 | 5 | low | 384 |
| Lemon cheesecake | 30 | 1 average slice | 13 | 5 | low | 273 |
| Lemon chicken | 3 | 1 average serving | 13 | 58 | 0 | 356 |
| Lemon curd | 9 | 1 level tbsp | 1 | trace | low | 42 |
| Lemon curd tart | 22 | 1 individual tart | 6 | 1 | low | 150 |
| Lemon danish pastry | 34 | 1 pastry | 13 | 4 | med | 263 |

| Food | Carbo-hydrate g | Portion size | Fat g | Protein g | Fibre | kCalories per portion |
|---|---|---|---|---|---|---|
| **Lemon drop cakes** | **20** | 1 individual cake | 5 | 1 | low | 130 |
| **Lemon drop sweets** (candies) | **5** | 1 sweet | 0 | 0 | 0 | 20 |
| **Lemon juice**, pure | **trace** | 1 tbsp | trace | trace | low | 1 |
| **Lemon meringue pie** | **50** | 1 slice | 16 | 5 | low | 362 |
| **Lemon mousse** | **38** | 1 average serving | 8 | 4 | low | 227 |
| **Lemon puffs** | **7** | 1 biscuit (cookie) | 4 | 1 | low | 69 |
| **Lemon sauce** | **10** | 2 level tbsp | 0 | trace | 0 | 43 |
| **Lemon sherbet sweets** (candies) | **5** | 1 sweet | 0 | 0 | 0 | 20 |
| **Lemon slice** | **19** | 1 cake | 5 | 1 | low | 125 |
| **Lemon sole**, fried (sautéed), in breadcrumbs | **15** | 1 medium fish | 21 | 25 | low | 342 |
| **Lemon sole, grilled (broiled)** | **0** | 1 medium fish | 4 | 25 | 0 | 158 |
| **Lemon sole, poached or steamed** | **0** | 1 medium fish | 1 | 29 | 0 | 128 |
| **Lemon sorbet** | **17** | 1 scoop | trace | trace | 0 | 65 |
| **Lemon soufflé** | **21** | 1 average serving | 41 | 6 | 0 | 315 |
| **Lemon sponge pudding** | **50** | 1 average serving | 11 | 3 | low | 308 |
| **Lemon squash**, diluted | **13** | 1 tumbler | trace | trace | 0 | 53 |
| **Lemon squash, low-calorie, diluted** | **trace** | 1 tumbler | 0 | trace | 0 | 2 |
| **Lemon tango** | **23** | 1 tumbler | trace | trace | 0 | 98 |

| Food | Carbo-hydrate g | Portion size | Fat g | Protein g | Fibre | kCalories per portion |
|---|---|---|---|---|---|---|
| Lemon tango, low-calorie | trace | 1 tumbler | trace | trace | 0 | 8 |
| **Lemon tea**, instant | 22 | 1 cup | 0 | trace | 0 | 88 |
| Lemon tea, instant, low-calorie | 1 | 1 cup | trace | trace | 0 | 5 |
| **Lemon water ice** | 17 | 1 scoop | trace | trace | 0 | 65 |
| **Lemonade**, home-made | 35 | 1 tumbler | trace | trace | 0 | 141 |
| Lemonade, sparkling | 11 | 1 tumbler | 0 | trace | 0 | 42 |
| Lemonade, sparkling, low-calorie | trace | 1 tumbler | 0 | 0 | 0 | 1 |
| **Lemonade shandy** | 14 | 1 tumbler | trace | 0 | low | 60 |
| **Lentil and bacon soup**, canned | 15 | 2 ladlefuls | 2 | 4 | med | 120 |
| **Lentil and bacon soup**, home-made | 26 | 2 ladlefuls | 51 | 14 | med | 302 |
| **Lentil and tomato soup**, canned | 20 | 2 ladlefuls | trace | 6 | med | 108 |
| **Lentil rissoles** | 15 | 1 rissole | 3 | 7 | high | 90 |
| **Lentil soup**, canned | 25 | 2 ladlefuls | 8 | 8 | med | 92 |
| Lentil soup, home-made | 26 | 2 ladlefuls | 8 | 9 | med | 198 |
| Lentil stew | 49 | 1 average serving | 2 | 19 | high | 282 |
| **Lentils**, green or brown, soaked and cooked | 17 | 3 heaped tbsp | 1 | 9 | high | 105 |
| Lentils, red, cooked | 17 | 3 heaped tbsp | trace | 8 | med | 100 |
| Lettuce | 1 | 1 good handful | 0 | trace | low | 2 |
| **Lettuce soup**, rich, home-made | 19 | 2 ladlefuls | 3 | 2 | low | 127 |

| Food | Carbo-hydrate g | Portion size | Fat g | Protein g | Fibre | kCalories per portion |
|---|---|---|---|---|---|---|
| **Light corn syrup** *See* Golden syrup | | | | | | |
| **Lilt**, pineapple and grapefruit | 23 | 1 tumbler | 0 | 0 | 0 | 90 |
| Lilt, pineapple and grapefruit, diet | 0 | 1 tumbler | 0 | 0 | 0 | 8 |
| **Lima beans** *See* Butter beans | | | | | | |
| **Limburger cheese** | trace | 1 small wedge | 8 | 6 | 0 | 93 |
| **Lime** | 1 | 1 fruit | 0 | trace | 0 | 9 |
| **Lime cordial**, diluted | 10 | 1 tumbler | trace | trace | 0 | 36 |
| **Lime pickle** | 2 | 1 level tbsp | 2 | trace | low | 23 |
| **Lime squash**, low-calorie, diluted | trace | 1 tumbler | 0 | trace | 0 | 2 |
| **Limeade** | 4 | 1 tumbler | 0 | trace | 0 | 16 |
| Limeade and lager | 13 | 1 tumbler | trace | trace | 0 | 54 |
| **Lincoln biscuits** (cookies) | 6 | 1 biscuit | 2 | trace | low | 43 |
| **Lincolnshire sausage**, grilled (broiled) | 3 | 1 sausage | 9 | 7 | low | 117 |
| **Ling**, grilled (broiled) | 0 | 1 piece of fillet | 1 | 37 | 0 | 168 |
| **Linguine** (pasta ribbons), dried, boiled | 51 | 1 average serving | 2 | 8 | med | 239 |
| Linguine, fresh, boiled | 57 | 1 average serving | 2 | 11 | med | 301 |
| **Lion bar**, chocolate | 20 | 1 standard bar | 6 | 1 | low | 145 |
| Lion bar, ice cream | 24 | 1 standard bar | 13 | 3 | low | 227 |

| Food | Carbo-hydrate g | Portion size | Fat g | Protein g | Fibre | kCalories per portion |
|---|---|---|---|---|---|---|
| **Liqueur coffee** | 7 | 1 wine glass | 14 | 1 | 0 | 218 |
| **Liquorice all-sorts** | 7 | 1 sweet (candy) | trace | trace | 0 | 29 |
| **Liquorice caramels** | 7 | 1 sweet (candy) | 1 | trace | 0 | 39 |
| **Liquorice sticks** | 1 | 1 stick | 0 | 0 | 0 | 5 |
| **Liver**, calves', braised | 3 | 3 medium slices | 7 | 22 | low | 165 |
| Liver, calves', fried (sautéed), in seasoned flour | 7 | 3 medium slices | 13 | 27 | 0 | 254 |
| Liver, lambs', fried (sautéed), in seasoned flour | 4 | 3 medium slices | 14 | 23 | 0 | 232 |
| Liver, pigs', stewed | 4 | 1 average serving | 8 | 26 | 0 | 189 |
| **Liver in seasoned flour and bacon**, fried (sautéed) | 8 | 1 average serving | 46 | 43 | 0 | 498 |
| **Liver and onions**, fried (sautéed) | 18 | 1 average serving | 25 | 25 | med | 396 |
| **Liver casserole** | 2 | 1 average serving | 9 | 31 | low | 220 |
| **Liver pâté** | 1 | 1 average serving | 14 | 6 | 0 | 158 |
| Liver pâté, en croûte | 24 | 1 med slice | 49 | 16 | low | 596 |
| Liver pâté, low-fat | 2 | 1 average serving | 10 | 7 | 0 | 131 |
| Liver pâté, with toast and butter | 35 | 1 average serving plus 2 slices of toast | 31 | 13 | med | 496 |
| **Liver sausage**, sliced | **trace** | 1 slice | 5 | 2 | 0 | 57 |
| Liver sausage, spreading | 1 | 1 level tbsp | 7 | 3 | low | 77 |
| **Livers**, chicken, fried (sautéed) | 3 | 1 average serving | 11 | 21 | 0 | 194 |

| Food | Carbo-hydrate g | Portion size | Fat g | Protein g | Fibre | kCalories per portion |
|------|------|------|------|------|------|------|
| **Lobster** | 0 | ½ med lobster | 4 | 24 | 0 | 126 |
| **Lobster bisque** | 10 | 2 ladlefuls | 4 | 13 | low | 108 |
| **Lobster mayonnaise salad** | 5 | ½ med lobster | 28 | 26 | high | 363 |
| **Lobster newburg** | 23 | 1 average serving | 5 | 20 | low | 225 |
| **Lobster salad** | 5 | ½ med lobster | 5 | 26 | high | 157 |
| **Lobster tails**, fried (sautéed), in breadcrumbs | 29 | 1 average serving | 18 | 12 | low | 316 |
| **Lobster thermidor** | 7 | ½ med lobster | 19 | 33 | 0 | 376 |
| **Lockets** | 41 | 1 tube | 0 | 0 | 0 | 165 |
| **Loganberries** | 13 | 3 heaped tbsp | trace | 1 | med | 55 |
| Loganberries, stewed | 11 | 3 heaped tbsp | trace | trace | med | 50 |
| Loganberries, stewed with sugar | 21 | 3 heaped tbsp | trace | trace | med | 80 |
| **Loquats** | 2 | 1 fruit | trace | trace | low | 7 |
| **Low-fat spread** | trace | 25 g/1 oz/2 tbsp | 12 | 3 | 0 | 117 |
| Low-fat spread | trace | 1 small knob | 4 | 1 | 0 | 39 |
| **Lucozade** | 36 | 1 tumbler | 0 | trace | 0 | 137 |
| **Lumachi** (pasta shapes), dried, boiled | 42 | 1 average serving | 1 | 7 | med | 198 |
| Lumachi, fresh, boiled | 45 | 1 average serving | 2 | 9 | med | 235 |
| **Lumpfish roe** | 1 | 1 level tbsp | 3 | 4 | 0 | 40 |
| **Lunch tongue** | trace | 1 med slice | 3 | 4 | 0 | 53 |
| **Luncheon meat** | 1 | 1 med slice | 9 | 4 | 0 | 100 |
| **Lychees** | 1 | 1 fruit | trace | trace | low | 5 |
| Lychees, canned in syrup | 18 | 3 heaped tbsp | trace | trace | low | 66 |
| **Lymeswold cheese** | trace | 1 small wedge | 10 | 4 | 0 | 106 |

| Food | Carbo-hydrate g | Portion size | Fat g | Protein g | Fibre | kCalories per portion |
|---|---|---|---|---|---|---|
| **M&Ms**, chocolate | 31 | 1 small bag | 1 | 2 | 0 | 219 |
| M&Ms, peanut | 26 | 1 small bag | 12 | 5 | low | 231 |
| **Macadamia nuts** | 1 | 1 small handful | 12 | 1 | high | 112 |
| **Macaroni**, dried, boiled | 42 | 1 average serving | 1 | 7 | med | 198 |
| Macaroni, fresh, boiled | 45 | 1 average serving | 1 | 9 | med | 235 |
| **Macaroni cheese** | 46 | 1 average serving | 17 | 23 | med | 436 |
| Macaroni cheese, canned | 19 | 1 small can | 10 | 7 | low | 188 |
| **Macaroons**, almond | 13 | 1 macaroon | 7 | 3 | med | 120 |
| Macaroons, coconut | 16 | 1 macaroon | 5 | 1 | med | 117 |
| **Macedoine** (mixed, diced vegetables), steamed or boiled | 7 | 3 heaped tbsp | trace | 3 | high | 42 |
| **Mackerel**, fried (sautéed) | 0 | 1 medium fish | 19 | 35 | 0 | 310 |
| Mackerel, grilled (broiled) | 0 | 1 medium fish | 15 | 38 | 0 | 279 |
| Mackerel, smoked | 0 | 1 medium fillet | 46 | 28 | 0 | 531 |
| Mackerel, smoked pâté | 0 | 1 average serving | 58 | 19 | 0 | 599 |
| Mackerel, soused | 6 | 1 roll | 9 | 16 | 0 | 165 |
| **Madeira**, dry | trace | 1 double measure | 0 | trace | 0 | 58 |
| Madeira, sweet | trace | 1 double measure | 0 | trace | 0 | 68 |
| **Madeira cake** | 58 | 1 average slice | 17 | 5 | low | 393 |
| **Madelaines** | 16 | 1 cake | 8 | 2 | low | 137 |
| **Magnum**, all flavours | 27 | 1 ice cream | 20 | 4 | 0 | 300 (average) |

| Food | Carbo-hydrate g | Portion size | Fat g | Protein g | Fibre | kCalories per portion |
|---|---|---|---|---|---|---|
| **Maids of honour** | 35 | 1 individual tart | 12 | 2 | low | 207 |
| **Maître d'hôtel butter** | trace | 1 level tbsp | 10 | trace | 0 | 92 |
| **Malt loaf** | 17 | 1 med slice | 1 | 2 | low | 80 |
| **Maltesers** | 18 | 1 small packet | 5 | 3 | 0 | 183 |
| **Mandarin orange** | 7 | 1 fruit | trace | 1 | med | 30 |
| Mandarin oranges, canned in natural juice | 8 | 3 heaped tbsp | trace | 1 | low | 32 |
| Mandarin oranges, canned in syrup | 13 | 3 heaped tbsp | trace | trace | low | 52 |
| **Mangetout** (snow peas) | 2 | 3 heaped tbsp | trace | 2 | med | 16 |
| Mangetout, steamed or boiled | 2 | 3 heaped tbsp | trace | 1 | med | 13 |
| Mangetout, stir-fried | 2 | 3 heaped tbsp | 2 | 2 | med | 35 |
| **Mango** | 24 | 1 medium fruit | trace | 1 | high | 97 |
| Mango, canned in syrup | 20 | 3 heaped tbsp | trace | trace | high | 77 |
| **Mango chutney** | 7 | 1 level tbsp | 2 | trace | low | 43 |
| **Mango mousse** | 18 | 1 average serving | 6 | 4 | low | 137 |
| **Mango sorbet** | 24 | 1 scoop | trace | trace | med | 88 |
| **Mangosteen** | 5 | 1 fruit | trace | trace | med | 20 |
| Mangosteen, canned in syrup | 18 | 3 heaped tbsp | trace | trace | med | 73 |
| **Maple syrup** | 15 | 1 level tbsp | 0 | 0 | 0 | 53 |
| **Maraschino cherries** | 3 | 1 fruit | trace | trace | low | 12 |
| **Maraschino liqueur** | 8 | 1 single measure | 0 | trace | 0 | 64 |

| Food | Carbo-hydrate g | Portion size | Fat g | Protein g | Fibre | kCalories per portion |
|---|---|---|---|---|---|---|
| **Marble cake** | 55 | 1 average slice | 14 | 5 | med | 371 |
| **Marc** | trace | 1 single measure | 0 | trace | 0 | 55 |
| **Margarine** | trace | 25 g/1 oz/2 tbsp | 20 | trace | 0 | 185 |
| Margarine | trace | 1 small knob | 8 | trace | 0 | 74 |
| **Margherita pizza,** Italian-style | 25 | 1 large slice | 12 | 9 | med | 235 |
| **Marie biscuits** (cookies) | 6 | 1 biscuit | 1 | trace | low | 35 |
| **Marlin steak,** fried (sautéed) | 0 | 1 medium steak | 14 | 44 | 0 | 294 |
| Marlin steak, grilled (broiled) | 0 | 1 med steak | 9 | 44 | 0 | 271 |
| **Marmalade** | 10 | 1 level tbsp | 0 | trace | low | 39 |
| Marmalade, reduced-sugar | 5 | 1 level tbsp | trace | trace | 0 | 21 |
| **Marmalade pudding** | 45 | 1 average serving | 16 | 6 | med | 340 |
| **Marmalade tart** | 46 | 1 average slice | 11 | 2 | med | 285 |
| **Marmite** | trace | 1 level tsp | trace | 2 | 0 | 9 |
| **Marrow** (squash), steamed or boiled | 2 | 3 heaped tbsp | trace | trace | low | 9 |
| Marrow, stuffed with meat | 38 | 1 large slice | 8 | 23 | low | 306 |
| **Marrowfat peas,** canned | 17 | 3 heaped tbsp | 1 | 7 | high | 100 |
| Marrowfat peas, soaked and boiled | 18 | 3 heaped tbsp | 1 | 6 | high | 82 |
| **Mars chocolate bar** | 45 | 1 standard bar | 11 | 3 | 0 | 294 |
| **Mars ice cream** | 22 | 1 standard bar | 12 | 3 | 0 | 209 |
| **Marsala** | 6 | 1 double measure | 0 | trace | 0 | 79 |

| Food | Carbo-hydrate g | Portion size | Fat g | Protein g | Fibre | kCalories per portion |
|---|---|---|---|---|---|---|
| **Mascarpone cheese** | trace | 1 good spoonful | 14 | trace | 0 | 128 |
| **Marshmallows** | 4 | 1 sweet (candy) | 0 | trace | 0 | 15 |
| **Marshmallow chocolate tea cakes** | 13 | 1 cake | 2 | 1 | low | 73 |
| **Martini**, dry | 3 | 1 double measure | 0 | trace | 0 | 59 |
| Martini, sweet | 8 | 1 double measure | 0 | trace | 0 | 75 |
| **Marzipan** | 17 | 25 g/1 oz | 4 | 1 | med | 101 |
| **Matchmakers** | 1 | 1 stick | trace | trace | 0 | 10 |
| **Matzos** | 23 | 1 cracker | trace | 3 | med | 100 |
| **Mayonnaise** | trace | 1 level tbsp | 11 | trace | 0 | 104 |
| Mayonnaise, low-calorie | 1 | 1 level tbsp | 4 | trace | 0 | 40 |
| **Mcchicken sandwich** | 39 | 1 sandwich | 17 | 16 | high | 375 |
| **Meat and potato pie** | 25 | 1 average serving | 19 | 24 | med | 330 |
| **Meat cobbler** | 40 | 1 average serving | 28 | 32 | high | 489 |
| **Meat paste** | 2 | 1 level tbsp | 3 | 1 | low | 35 |
| **Meat pie** | 32 | 1 individual pie | 28 | 18 | low | 460 |
| **Meatballs**, fried (sautéed) | 0 | 4 meatballs | 15 | 28 | 0 | 246 |
| Meatballs, grilled (broiled) | 0 | 4 meatballs | 12 | 27 | 0 | 218 |
| **Meatballs in gravy**, canned | 9 | ½ large can | 14 | 11 | low | 208 |
| **Meatballs in tomato sauce**, canned | 33 | ½ large can | 7 | 8 | med | 227 |

| Food | Carbo-hydrate g | Portion size | Fat g | Protein g | Fibre | kCalories per portion |
|---|---|---|---|---|---|---|
| **Meatballs with spaghetti** | 80 | 1 average serving | 31 | 36 | med | 718 |
| **Meatloaf** | 10 | 1 thick slice | 9 | 21 | low | 208 |
| Meatloaf, with tomato sauce | 22 | 2 slices | 18 | 30 | med | 370 |
| **Mediterranean vegetables,** roasted | 10 | 1 average serving | 5 | 1 | high | 80 |
| **Melba toast** | 11 | 1 slice | trace | 2 | low | 53 |
| **Melon** *See individual varieties, e.g.* Cantaloupe melon | | | | | | |
| **Melon cocktail** | 12 | 1 average serving | trace | 1 | low | 48 |
| **Melon with parma ham** | 15 | 1 slice of melon +2 slices of ham | 1 | 9 | low | 105 |
| **Melton Mowbray pork pie** | 45 | 1 standard pie | 48 | 18 | med | 677 |
| **Meringue** | 24 | 1 meringue | trace | 1 | 0 | 95 |
| Meringue, with cream | 24 | 1 meringue | 7 | 1 | 0 | 162 |
| **Meringue nest,** with fresh fruit | 32 | 1 meringue | 1 | 3 | med | 141 |
| **Milk loaf** | 12 | 1 med slice | 1 | 2 | low | 60 |
| **Milk powder,** dried (non-fat dried milk) | 8 | 1 level tbsp | trace | 5 | 0 | 52 |
| **Milk,** Channel Island | 14 | 300 ml/½ pt/ 1¼ cups | 15 | 11 | 0 | 234 |
| Milk, condensed, skimmed, sweetened | 60 | 100 ml/3½ fl oz/ scant ½ cup | trace | 10 | 0 | 267 |

| Food | Carbo-hydrate g | Portion size | Fat g | Protein g | Fibre | kCalories per portion |
|---|---|---|---|---|---|---|
| Milk, condensed, whole, sweetened | 55 | 100 ml/3½ fl oz/ scant ½ cup | 10 | 8 | 0 | 333 |
| Milk, condensed, skimmed, unsweetened | 11 | 100 ml/3½ fl oz/ scant ½ cup | trace | 10 | 0 | 80 |
| Milk, condensed, whole, unsweetened | 8 | 100 ml/3½ fl oz/ scant ½ cup | 9 | 8 | 0 | 151 |
| Milk, semi-skimmed | 15 | 300 ml/½ pt/ 1¼ cups | 5 | 10 | 0 | 138 |
| Milk, skimmed | 15 | 300 ml/½ pt/ 1¼ cups | trace | 10 | 0 | 99 |
| Milk, whole | 14 | 300 ml/½ pt/ 1¼ cups | 12 | 10 | 0 | 198 |
| **Milk chocolate** | 28 | 1 standard bar | 14 | 4 | 0 | 255 |
| **Milk classico** ice lolly | 9 | 1 lolly | 13 | 2 | 0 | 141 |
| **Milk jelly** (jello), made with semi-skimmed milk | 28 | 1 average serving | 2 | 6 | 0 | 148 |
| Milk jelly, made with skimmed milk | 28 | 1 average serving | trace | 6 | 0 | 132 |
| **Milkshake**, extra-thick | 42 | 1 tumbler | 5 | 6 | low | 238 |
| Milkshake, made with granules and semi-skimmed milk | 23 | 1 tumbler | 3 | 6 | low | 138 |
| Milkshake, made with granules and skimmed milk | 23 | 1 tumbler | trace | 6 | low | 109 |

| Food | Carbo-hydrate g | Portion size | Fat g | Protein g | Fibre | kCalories per portion |
|---|---|---|---|---|---|---|
| Milkshake, made with syrup and semi-skimmed milk | 18 | 1 tumbler | 3 | 7 | low | 125 |
| Milkshake, made with syrup and skimmed milk | 18 | 1 tumbler | trace | 7 | low | 106 |
| **Milk stick** | 24 | 1 lolly | 18 | 3 | 0 | 275 |
| **Milky bar** chocolate bar | 17 | 1 standard bar | 9 | 2 | 0 | 163 |
| **Milky way** chocolate bar | 19 | 1 standard bar | 4 | 1 | 0 | 117 |
| Milky way crispy rolls | 14 | 1 roll | 7 | 2 | low | 131 |
| **Millet flakes** | 19 | 25 g/1 oz/¼ cup | trace | 1 | med | 80 |
| **Mince** See *individual meats, e.g.* Beef, minced | | | | | | |
| **Mince pie**, sweet | 39 | 1 individual pie | 9 | 2 | low | 244 |
| **Mincemeat** | 9 | 1 level tbsp | 1 | trace | low | 41 |
| **Minestrone**, canned | 15 | 2 ladlefuls | 1 | 3 | med | 85 |
| Minestrone, home-made | 39 | 2 ladlefuls | 7 | 10 | high | 248 |
| Minestrone, packet | 15 | 2 ladlefuls | 2 | 1 | med | 79 |
| **Minibix with chocolate**, dry | 18 | 25 g/1 oz/½ cup | 1 | 2 | med | 96 |
| Minibix with chocolate, with semi-skimmed milk | 35 | 3 heaped tbsp | 4 | 7 | med | 212 |
| Minibix with chocolate, with skimmed milk | 35 | 3 heaped tbsp | 3 | 7 | med | 196 |

| Food | Carbo-hydrate g | Portion size | Fat g | Protein g | Fibre | kCalories per portion |
|---|---|---|---|---|---|---|
| Minstrels | 29 | 1 small packet | 9 | 2 | 0 | 206 |
| Mint chocolate chip ice cream | 12 | 1 scoop | 4 | 2 | low | 91 |
| Mint imperials | 5 | 1 sweet (candy) | 0 | 0 | 0 | 18 |
| Mint jelly (clear conserve) | 6 | 1 level tbsp | trace | trace | 0 | 38 |
| Mint sauce | 4 | 1 level tbsp | trace | trace | 0 | 18 |
| Miso soup, Japanese | 8 | 1 average serving | 4 | 5 | med | 78 |
| Mississippi mud pie | 38 | 1 average slice | 18 | 5 | low | 325 |
| Mivi ice lolly, all flavours | 13 | 1 lolly | 3 | 1 | 0 | 83 (average) |
| Mixed (candied) peel | 9 | 1 level tbsp | trace | trace | low | 35 |
| Mixed salad | 5 | 1 average serving | 1 | 2 | high | 31 |
| Mixed salad, dressed | 5 | 1 average serving | 18 | 2 | high | 128 |
| Molasses | 10 | 1 level tbsp | 0 | trace | 0 | 38 |
| Monkey nuts, raw, shelled See also Peanuts | 2 | 1 small handful | 7 | 4 | high | 85 |
| Monkfish, grilled (broiled) | 0 | 1 piece of fillet | 3 | 31 | 0 | 170 |
| Monkfish, roasted | 0 | 1 piece of fillet | 7 | 31 | low | 216 |
| Monkfish stew | 43 | 1 average serving | 5 | 30 | med | 330 |
| Monterey jack cheese | trace | 1 small wedge | 9 | 7 | 0 | 106 |
| Morning rolls | 29 | 1 roll | 2 | 5 | low | 140 |
| Mortadella | trace | 1 med slice | 4 | 2 | 0 | 47 |
| Moules à la crème | 11 | 1 average serving | 21 | 21 | low | 372 |

| Food | Carbo-hydrate g | Portion size | Fat g | Protein g | Fibre | kCalories per portion |
|------|------|------|------|------|------|------|
| **Moules à la marinière** | **11** | 1 average serving | 7 | 21 | low | 238 |
| **Moussaka** | **21** | 1 average serving | 41 | 27 | med | 552 |
| **Mozzarella cheese**, Danish | **trace** | 1 thick slice | 5 | 6 | 0 | 77 |
| Mozzarella cheese, Italian | **1** | ¼ round cheese | 6 | 5 | 0 | 80 |
| **Muesli**, dry | **16** | 25 g/1 oz/¼ cup | 2 | 2 | high | 91 |
| Muesli, with semi-skimmed milk | **33** | 3 heaped tbsp | 5 | 8 | high | 203 |
| Muesli, with skimmed milk | **33** | 3 heaped tbsp | 3 | 8 | high | 189 |
| **Muffin**, American | **24** | 1 muffin | 6 | 4 | med | 169 |
| Muffin, English | **25** | 1 muffin | 1 | 5 | med | 127 |
| Muffin, English, toasted, with butter | **25** | 1 muffin | 8 | 5 | med | 200 |
| Muffin, English, toasted, with low-fat spread | **25** | 1 muffin | 5 | 6 | med | 166 |
| **Mulberries** | **10** | 3 heaped tbsp | trace | 1 | med | 43 |
| **Mulled wine** | **5** | 1 wine glass | 0 | trace | 0 | 105 |
| **Mullet**, grey or red, grilled (broiled) | **0** | 1 medium fillet | 4 | 23 | 0 | 139 |
| **Mulligatawny soup**, canned | **13** | 2 ladlefuls | 7 | 4 | med | 137 |
| **Multi-grain start**, dry | **20** | 25 g/1 oz/½ cup | trace | 2 | med | 90 |
| Multi-grain start, with semi-skimmed milk | **38** | 5 heaped tbsp | 3 | 7 | med | 201 |

| Food | Carbo-hydrate g | Portion size | Fat g | Protein g | Fibre | kCalories per portion |
|---|---|---|---|---|---|---|
| Multi-grain start, with skimmed milk | 38 | 5 heaped tbsp | 1 | 7 | med | 185 |
| Munchies | 3 | 1 sweet | 1 | trace | 0 | 22 |
| Mung beans, dried, soaked and cooked | 18 | 3 heaped tbsp | trace | 7 | high | 105 |
| Mung beans, sprouted | 1 | 1 good handful | trace | trace | high | 6 |
| Mung beans, sprouted, canned | 2 | 3 heaped tbsp | trace | 1 | high | 12 |
| Munster cheese | trace | 1 small wedge | 8 | 7 | 0 | 104 |
| Muscatels, stoned (pitted) | 10 | 1 small handful | trace | trace | low | 41 |
| Mushroom bhaji | 9 | 1 bhaji | 8 | 3 | med | 123 |
| Mushroom ketchup | trace | 1 level tsp | trace | trace | 0 | 6 |
| Mushroom omelette | trace | 2 eggs | 26 | 14 | low | 295 |
| Mushroom pâté | 4 | ½ small tub | 9 | 3 | 0 | 117 |
| Mushroom pâté, home-made | 1 | 1 average serving | 19 | 1 | low | 191 |
| Mushroom and cheese quiche | 18 | 1 large slice | 26 | 14 | low | 353 |
| Mushroom ragu | 3 | 1 average serving | 30 | 4 | low | 311 |
| Mushroom risotto | 52 | 1 average serving | 14 | 5 | low | 341 |
| Mushroom pasta sauce | 7 | ¼ jar | 10 | trace | 0 | 45 |
| Mushroom sauce, made with semi-skimmed milk | 8 | 5 level tbsp | 6 | 3 | low | 99 |

| Food | Carbo-hydrate g | Portion size | Fat g | Protein g | Fibre | kCalories per portion |
|---|---|---|---|---|---|---|
| Mushroom sauce, made with skimmed milk | 8 | 5 level tbsp | 5 | 3 | low | 89 |
| **Mushroom soup,** cream of, canned | 8 | 2 ladlefuls | 8 | 2 | 0 | 106 |
| Mushroom soup, home-made | 14 | 2 ladlefuls | 2 | 7 | low | 156 |
| Mushroom soup, low-fat, canned | 7 | 2 ladlefuls | 1 | 2 | low | 48 |
| Mushroom soup, instant | 13 | 1 mug | 5 | trace | 0 | 96 |
| Mushroom soup, packet | 21 | 2 ladlefuls | 2 | 4 | 0 | 118 |
| **Mushrooms** *See also individual types, e.g.* Shiitake mushrooms | trace | 1 med mushroom | trace | trace | low | 2 |
| Mushrooms, breaded | 8 | 1 average serving | 16 | 3 | med | 196 |
| Mushrooms, button, sliced and fried (sautéed) | trace | 2 good tbsp | 8 | 1 | med | 78 |
| Mushrooms, large, flat, fried | trace | 2 large | 16 | 2 | med | 157 |
| Mushrooms, stewed | trace | 2 good tbsp | trace | 1 | med | 5 |
| Mushrooms, stuffed | 4 | 1 large | 2 | 2 | low | 53 |
| **Mushrooms à la grecque** | 4 | 1 average serving | 30 | 2 | low | 171 |
| **Mushy peas,** canned | 16 | 3 heaped tbsp | trace | 6 | high | 69 |
| **Mussels,** cooked, shelled | trace | 1 mussel | trace | trace | 0 | 3 |

| Food | Carbo-hydrate g | Portion size | Fat g | Protein g | Fibre | kCalories per portion |
|------|------|------|------|------|------|------|
| Mussels, smoked, canned, drained *See also* Moules | 2 | ½ small can | 5 | 2 | 0 | 96 |
| Mustard *See individual varieties, e.g.* Dijon mustard | | | | | | |
| **Mustard and cress** | trace | 1 good spoonful | trace | trace | med | 2 |
| **Mustard butter** | trace | 1 level tbsp | 6 | trace | 0 | 118 |
| **Mustard chicken** | 3 | 1 med breast | 5 | 26 | 0 | 176 |
| **Mustard sauce**, made with semi-skimmed milk | 8 | 5 level tbsp | 6 | 3 | low | 103 |
| Mustard sauce, made with skimmed milk | 8 | 5 level tbsp | 5 | 3 | low | 93 |
| **Mutton**, boiled | 0 | 2 thick slices | 16 | 28 | 0 | 253 |
| **Mutton, haricot** | 24 | 1 average serving | 9 | 21 | med | 252 |
| **Mutton pie** | 24 | 1 individual pie | 5 | 8 | med | 225 |
| **Mutton stew** | 24 | 1 average serving | 21 | 14 | med | 369 |

| Food | Carbo-hydrate g | Portion size | Fat g | Protein g | Fibre | kCalories per portion |
|---|---|---|---|---|---|---|
| **Naan bread**, plain | 29 | 1 small bread | 4 | 6 | med | 175 |
| **Nachos with cheese** | 36 | 6 pieces | 19 | 9 | low | 346 |
| **Napoletana pizza** | 25 | 1 large slice | 13 | 10 | med | 247 |
| **Napoletana sauce** | 9 | ¼ jar | 2 | 2 | low | 61 |
| **Navy beans** *See* Haricot beans | | | | | | |
| **Neapolitan ice cream** | 10 | 1 scoop | 4 | 2 | 0 | 86 |
| **Nectarine** | 12 | 1 fruit | trace | 2 | med | 52 |
| **Nesquick cereal**, dry | 21 | 25 g/1 oz/½ cup | 1 | 1 | low | 98 |
| **Nesquick cereal, with** semi-skimmed milk | 31 | 5 heaped tbsp | 3 | 5 | low | 179 |
| **Nesquick cereal, with** skimmed milk | 31 | 5 heaped tbsp | 1 | 5 | low | 163 |
| **Nesquick milk shake flavouring** *See* Milkshakes | | | | | | |
| **Neufchatel cheese** | 1 | 1 small wedge | 7 | 3 | 0 | 74 |
| **Nice biscuits** (cookies) | 5 | 1 biscuit | 1 | trace | low | 35 |
| **Niçoise salad** | 34 | 1 average serving | 11 | 21 | high | 308 |
| **Noilly prat** | 3 | 1 double measure | 0 | trace | 0 | 59 |
| **Noisettes of lamb,** grilled (broiled) | 0 | 2 noisettes | 12 | 28 | 0 | 222 |
| **Noodles**, dried, boiled | 51 | 1 average serving | 2 | 8 | med | 239 |

| Food | Carbo-hydrate g | Portion size | Fat g | Protein g | Fibre | kCalories per portion |
|------|------|------|------|------|------|------|
| Noodles, fresh, boiled *See also individual types, e.g.* Chinese egg noodles | 57 | 1 average serving | 2 | 11 | med | 301 |
| Norwegian apple cake | 32 | 1 average slice | 10 | 3 | high | 252 |
| Norwegian blue cheese | trace | 1 small wedge | 7 | 5 | 0 | 87 |
| Norwegian cream | 25 | 1 average serving | 79 | 6 | 0 | 835 |
| Nut brittle | 34 | 1 standard bar | 9 | 3 | med | 226 |
| Nut cutlet | 5 | 1 cutlet | 10 | 5 | med | 139 |
| Nut rissole | 6 | 1 rissole | 18 | 7 | med | 203 |
| Nut roast | 13 | 1 average serving | 29 | 12 | high | 366 |
| Nutri-grain breakfast bars, all flavours | 24 | 1 bar | 3 | 1 | med | 130 (average) |
| Nuts *See individual varieties, e.g.* brazil nuts | | | | | | |
| Nuts, mixed | 2 | 25 g/1 oz/¼ cup | 13 | 6 | high | 151 |
| Nuts and raisins | 7 | 1 small handful | 7 | 3 | high | 108 |

| Food | Carbo-hydrate g | Portion size | Fat g | Protein g | Fibre | kCalories per portion |
|------|------|------|------|------|------|------|
| **Oat bran** | 9 | 1 level tbsp | 1 | 2 | high | 51 |
| **Oat bran crispbread** | 5 | 1 crispbread | trace | 1 | med | 27 |
| **Oat bran flakes**, dry | 16 | 25 g/1 oz/½ cup | 1 | 2 | high | 87 |
| Oat bran flakes, with semi-skimmed milk | 33 | 5 heaped tbsp | 4 | 8 | high | 197 |
| Oat bran flakes, with skimmed milk | 33 | 5 heaped tbsp | 2 | 8 | high | 181 |
| **Oat cereal**, instant *See* Ready brek | | | | | | |
| **Oat flakes**, dry | 17 | 25 g/1 oz/½ cup | 18 | 3 | high | 96 |
| Oat flakes, with semi-skimmed milk | 33 | 5 heaped tbsp | 5 | 9 | high | 211 |
| Oat flakes, with skimmed milk | 33 | 5 heaped tbsp | 3 | 9 | high | 195 |
| Oat krunchies, dry | 19 | 25 g/1 oz/½ cup | 1 | 2 | med | 98 |
| Oat krunchies, with semi-skimmed milk | 25 | 5 heaped tbsp | 3 | 6 | med | 214 |
| Oat krunchies, with skimmed milk | 25 | 5 heaped tbsp | 1 | 6 | med | 198 |
| **Oatcakes** | 8 | 1 oatcake | 2 | 1 | med | 59 |
| **Oatmeal** | 16 | 25 g/1 oz/¼ cup | 2 | 3 | med | 94 |
| **Oatmeal porridge**, made with semi-skimmed milk | 32 | 1 average serving | 6 | 11 | med | 207 |
| Oatmeal porridge, made with skimmed milk | 32 | 1 average serving | 6 | 11 | med | 191 |
| Oatmeal porridge, made with water | 26 | 1 average serving | 4 | 4 | med | 150 |

| Food | Carbo-hydrate g | Portion size | Fat g | Protein g | Fibre | kCalories per portion |
|---|---|---|---|---|---|---|
| **Oats**, rolled | 18 | 25 g/1 oz/¼ cup | 1 | 3 | med | 100 |
| Oats, rolled, porridge, made with semi-skimmed milk | 35 | 1 average serving | 6 | 9 | med | 217 |
| Oats, rolled, porridge, made with skimmed milk | 35 | 1 average serving | 4 | 9 | med | 201 |
| Oats, rolled, porridge, made with water | 29 | 1 average serving | 4 | 5 | med | 160 |
| **Octopus** | 4 | 1 average serving | 2 | 30 | 0 | 164 |
| Octopus, marinated in olive oil | 2 | ½ small can | 16 | 12 | 0 | 200 |
| **Ogen melon** | 13 | ½ melon | trace | 2 | med | 57 |
| **Oil**, all types | 0 | 1 tbsp | 15 | trace | 0 | 135 |
| **Okra** (ladies' fingers), steamed or boiled | 3 | 3 heaped tbsp | 1 | 2 | high | 28 |
| Okra, stir-fried | 4 | 3 heaped tbsp | 26 | 4 | high | 269 |
| **Olives**, black or green | trace | 1 olive | 1 | trace | med | 7 |
| Olives, stuffed | trace | 1 olive | trace | trace | med | 4 |
| Olives, with feta cheese | trace | 1 piece of each | 2 | 1 | low | 19 |
| **Omelette** *See also individual fillings, e.g. Cheese omelette* | trace | 2 eggs | 22 | 14 | 0 | 256 |
| **Omelette Arnold Bennett** | trace | 2 eggs | 29 | 25 | 0 | 373 |
| **Onion** | 8 | 1 medium onion | trace | 1 | med | 36 |

| Food | Carbo-hydrate g | Portion size | Fat g | Protein g | Fibre | kCalories per portion |
|---|---|---|---|---|---|---|
| Onion, fried (sautéed) | 7 | 2 good tbsp | 5 | 1 | med | 82 |
| Onion, pickled | 1 | 1 onion | trace | trace | low | 4 |
| Onion, spring (scallion) | trace | 1 onion | trace | trace | low | 3 |
| Onion, stuffed | 19 | 1 large onion | 8 | 13 | high | 190 |
| Onion bhaji | 9 | 1 bhaji | 8 | 3 | med | 123 |
| Onion dip | 1 | 2 level tbsp | 1 | 4 | 0 | 27 |
| Onion pakoras | 9 | 1 pakora | 11 | 3 | med | 148 |
| Onion rings, deep-fried in batter or breadcrumbs | 9 | 5 rings | 6 | 1 | low | 97 |
| Onion sauce, made with semi-skimmed milk | 6 | 5 level tbsp | 4 | 2 | low | 64 |
| Onion sauce, made with skimmed milk | 6 | 5 level tbsp | 3 | 2 | low | 55 |
| Onion soup, cream of canned | 8 | 2 ladlefuls | 6 | 1 | low | 88 |
| Onion soup, French, home-made | 8 | 2 ladlefuls | 6 | 2 | low | 94 |
| Onion soup, French, packet | 20 | 2 ladlefuls | 1 | 2 | low | 104 |
| Onion soup, French, with cheese croûte | 21 | 2 ladlefuls plus 1 croûte | 8 | 9 | low | 226 |
| Onion soup, white, home-made | 12 | 2 ladlefuls | 3 | 6 | low | 121 |
| Onion soup, white, packet | 4 | 2 ladlefuls | trace | trace | low | 77 |
| Onions in white sauce | 6 | 3 heaped tbsp | 1 | 1 | high | 36 |

| Food | Carbo-hydrate g | Portion size | Fat g | Protein g | Fibre | kCalories per portion |
|---|---|---|---|---|---|---|
| **Orange** | **13** | 1 fruit | 1 | 6 | med | 57 |
| **Orange and pineapple pure fruit juice** | **22** | 1 tumbler | trace | 1 | 0 | 84 |
| **Orange and pineapple squash**, diluted | **22** | 1 tumbler | trace | trace | 0 | 96 |
| Orange and pineapple squash, low-calorie, diluted | **5** | 1 tumbler | trace | trace | 0 | 22 |
| **Orange barley water**, diluted | **10** | 1 tumbler | trace | trace | 0 | 40 |
| **Orange cake** | **32** | 1 average slice | 17 | 2 | low | 290 |
| **Orange curd** | **9** | 1 level tbsp | 1 | trace | low | 42 |
| **Orange ice lolly** | **19** | 1 lolly | 0 | trace | 0 | 78 |
| **Orange jelly** (jello), fresh | **7** | 1 average serving | 0 | 3 | low | 40 |
| **Orange mousse** | **18** | 1 average serving | 6 | 4 | low | 137 |
| **Orange pure fruit juice** | **14** | 1 tumbler | trace | 1 | low | 72 |
| **Orange sauce** | **10** | 2 level tbsp | trace | trace | 0 | 40 |
| **Orange squash**, diluted | **22** | 1 tumbler | trace | trace | 0 | 96 |
| Orange squash, low-calorie, diluted | **5** | 1 tumbler | trace | 0 | 0 | 24 |
| **Orange tango** | **25** | 1 tumbler | 0 | 0 | 0 | 92 |
| Orange tango, low-calorie | **2** | 1 tumbler | trace | trace | 0 | 9 |
| **Orange water ice** | **16** | 1 scoop | 0 | trace | 0 | 64 |
| **Orangeade**, sparkling | **4** | 1 tumbler | 0 | 0 | 0 | 20 |

| Food | Carbo-hydrate g | Portion size | Fat g | Protein g | Fibre | kCalories per portion |
|---|---|---|---|---|---|---|
| **Oranges in caramel** | 33 | 1 average serving | 1 | 6 | med | 139 |
| **Original crunchy cereal**, dry | 16 | 25 g/1 oz/¼ cup | 3 | 2 | high | 97 |
| Original crunchy cereal, with semi-skimmed milk | 37 | 3 heaped tbsp | 7 | 9 | high | 250 |
| Original crunchy cereal, with skimmed milk | 37 | 3 heaped tbsp | 5 | 9 | high | 234 |
| **Osso buco** | 17 | 1 average serving | 10 | 55 | low | 382 |
| **Ovaltine**, made with semi-skimmed milk | 32 | 1 mug | 4 | 10 | low | 197 |
| Ovaltine, made with skimmed milk | 32 | 1 mug | trace | 10 | low | 165 |
| Ovaltine light, instant, made with water | 13 | 1 mug | 1 | 2 | low | 72 |
| **Oven chips** (fries) *See* Chips | | | | | | |
| **Ox tongue**, sliced | 0 | 1 medium slice | 6 | 5 | 0 | 73 |
| **Oxo** | 4 | 1 cube | trace | 2 | 0 | 27 |
| **Oxo drink** | trace | 1 mug | 0 | 2 | 0 | 10 |
| **Oxtail soup**, canned | 10 | 2 ladlefuls | 3 | 5 | 0 | 88 |
| Oxtail soup, instant | 14 | 1 mug | 2 | 1 | 0 | 77 |
| Oxtail soup, packet | 8 | 2 ladlefuls | 2 | 3 | 0 | 54 |
| **Oxtail and vegetable stew** | 7 | 1 average serving | 15 | 38 | high | 318 |

| Food | Carbo-hydrate g | Portion size | Fat g | Protein g | Fibre | kCalories per portion |
|---|---|---|---|---|---|---|
| **Oyster mushrooms** | **trace** | 1 mushroom | trace | trace | low | 1 |
| Oyster mushrooms, fried (sautéed) | **trace** | 2 good tbsp | 8 | 1 | low | 77 |
| Oyster mushrooms, stewed | **trace** | 2 good tbsp | trace | 1 | low | 3 |
| **Oysters** | **trace** | 1 oyster | trace | 1 | 0 | 7 |
| Oysters, fried (sautéed), in batter | **40** | 6 oysters | 18 | 12 | low | 368 |
| Oysters, smoked, canned, drained | **trace** | ½ small can | 6 | 9 | 0 | 103 |

| Food | Carbo-hydrate g | Portion size | Fat g | Protein g | Fibre | kCalories per portion |
|---|---|---|---|---|---|---|
| **Paella**, dried | 55 | 1 average serving | 3 | 11 | low | 294 |
| Paella, home-made | 34 | 1 average serving | 11 | 40 | low | 411 |
| **Pain au chocolat** | 26 | 1 pastry | 13 | 4 | low | 236 |
| **Pain au raisin** | 27 | 1 pastry | 10 | 4 | med | 212 |
| **Pain perdu** | 17 | 1 medium slice | 18 | 6 | low | 213 |
| **Pak choi/soi** | 2 | 1 head | trace | 1 | med | 19 |
| Pak choi/soi, steamed or boiled | 2 | 3 heaped tbsp | trace | 1 | med | 12 |
| Pak choi/soi, stir-fried | 2 | 3 heaped tbsp | 2 | 1 | med | 36 |
| **Pakora** | 9 | 1 pakora | 11 | 3 | med | 148 |
| **Palm hearts**, canned, drained | 2 | 1 piece | trace | 1 | low | 9 |
| **Palmiers** | 12 | 1 palmier | 6 | 1 | low | 83 |
| **Pancake**, buckwheat | 6 | 1 pancake | 2 | 2 | low | 45 |
| Pancake, potato | 22 | 1 pancake | 11 | 5 | med | 207 |
| Pancake, scotch | 6 | 1 pancake | 2 | 1 | low | 44 |
| Pancake, wheat *See also* Crêpe *and* Drop scone | 8 | 1 pancake | 6 | 2 | low | 100 |
| Pancake, with lemon and sugar | 13 | 1 pancake | 6 | 2 | low | 120 |
| **Pancake roll**, large | 21 | 1 large roll | 12 | 7 | low | 217 |
| Pancake roll, small | 7 | 1 small roll | 3 | 3 | low | 70 |
| **Pancetta**, diced, fried (sautéed) | 0 | 2 level tbsp | 22 | 11 | 0 | 248 |
| **Panna cotta** | 38 | 1 average serving | 17 | 2 | low | 328 |

| Food | Carbo-hydrate g | Portion size | Fat g | Protein g | Fibre | kCalories per portion |
|------|-----------------|--------------|-------|-----------|-------|------------------------|
| **Pappardelle** (pasta ribbons), dried, boiled | 51 | 1 average serving | 2 | 8 | med | 239 |
| Pappardelle, fresh, boiled | 57 | 1 average serving | 2 | 11 | med | 301 |
| **Papaya** | 30 | 1 medium fruit | trace | 2 | high | 118 |
| Papaya, canned in natural juice | 17 | 3 heaped tbsp | trace | trace | low | 65 |
| **Paratha** | 62 | 1 paratha | 20 | 12 | high | 450 |
| **Parkin** | 29 | 1 average piece | 7 | 2 | low | 185 |
| **Parma ham** | 0 | 1 thin slice | 1 | 4 | 0 | 21 |
| Parma ham, with figs | 11 | 1 fig plus 2 slices of ham | 2 | 9 | med | 87 |
| Parma ham, with melon | 15 | 1 slice of melon + 2 slices of ham | 1 | 9 | low | 105 |
| **Parmesan cheese** | trace | 1 small chunk | 8 | 10 | 0 | 113 |
| Parmesan cheese, grated | trace | 1 level tbsp | 5 | 6 | 0 | 68 |
| **Parsley sauce**, made with semi-skimmed milk | 8 | 5 level tbsp | 6 | 3 | low | 99 |
| Parsley sauce, made with skimmed milk | 8 | 5 level tbsp | 5 | 3 | low | 89 |
| **Parsnip** | 22 | 1 medium parsnip | 2 | 3 | high | 112 |
| Parsnip, roasted | 22 | 4 pieces | 6 | 3 | high | 156 |
| Parsnip, steamed or boiled | 13 | 1 average serving | 1 | 2 | high | 66 |
| **Partridge**, roast | 0 | ½ small bird | 7 | 37 | 0 | 212 |
| **Passata** (sieved tomatoes) | 6 | 5 level tbsp | trace | 1 | 0 | 29 |

| Food | Carbo-hydrate g | Portion size | Fat g | Protein g | Fibre | kCalories per portion |
|---|---|---|---|---|---|---|
| **Passion fruit** | 4 | 1 fruit | trace | trace | med | 17 |
| **Passion fruit ice cream** | 11 | 1 scoop | 3 | 1 | 0 | 83 |
| **Pasta salad** | 28 | 1 average serving | 8 | 5 | high | 197 |
| **Pasta sauce,** traditional, ready-made *See also individual flavours, e.g.* Tomato and herb | 8 | ¼ jar | 2 | 3 | 0 | 58 |
| **Pasta shapes,** dried, boiled | 42 | 1 average serving | 1 | 7 | med | 198 |
| Pasta shapes, fresh, boiled | 45 | 1 average serving | 2 | 9 | med | 235 |
| Pasta shapes, wholemeal, dried, boiled | 44 | 1 average serving | 2 | 10 | high | 218 |
| **Pasta strands**, all sizes, dried, boiled | 51 | 1 average serving | 2 | 8 | med | 239 |
| Pasta strands, fresh, boiled | 57 | 1 average serving | 2 | 11 | med | 301 |
| Pasta strands, wholemeal, dried, boiled | 152 | 1 average serving | 6 | 31 | high | 259 |
| **Pastis** | trace | 1 single measure | 0 | trace | 0 | 61 |
| **Pastrami** | 1 | 1 medium slice | 8 | 5 | 0 | 99 |
| Pastrami, on rye bread | 12 | 1 slice of each | 8 | 7 | med | 154 |
| **Pâté**, with toast and butter | 35 | 1 average serving +2 slices of toast | 31 | 13 | med | 496 |

| Food | Carbo-hydrate g | Portion size | Fat g | Protein g | Fibre | kCalories per portion |
|---|---|---|---|---|---|---|
| **Pavlova**, topped with cream and fruit | 45 | 1 average serving | 14 | 5 | med | 320 |
| **Paw paw** | 30 | 1 medium fruit | trace | 2 | high | 118 |
| **Pea and ham soup**, canned | 19 | 2 ladlefuls | 6 | 6 | high | 150 |
| Pea and ham soup, packet | 18 | 2 ladlefuls | 7 | 3 | med | 150 |
| Pea soup, canned | 30 | 2 ladlefuls | 6 | 10 | med | 188 |
| Pea soup, instant | 16 | 1 mug | 2 | 2 | med | 95 |
| **Peach** | 11 | 1 peach | trace | 1 | med | 42 |
| **Peach and apple pure fruit juice** | 20 | 1 tumbler | trace | 1 | low | 84 |
| **Peach chutney** | 6 | 1 level tbsp | trace | trace | low | 24 |
| **Peach melba** | 28 | 1 average serving | 5 | 3 | med | 169 |
| **Peach pie** | 38 | 1 average slice | 12 | 2 | low | 261 |
| **Peach squash**, diluted | 22 | 1 tumbler | trace | trace | 0 | 96 |
| Peach squash, low-calorie, diluted | 5 | 1 tumbler | trace | 0 | 0 | 24 |
| **Peaches**, dried | 8 | 1 piece | trace | trace | high | 31 |
| Peaches, dried, stewed | 20 | 3 heaped tbsp | trace | 1 | high | 77 |
| Peaches, dried, stewed with sugar | 27 | 3 heaped tbsp | trace | 1 | high | 103 |
| Peaches, sliced, canned in natural juice | 10 | 3 heaped tbsp | trace | 1 | low | 39 |
| Peaches, sliced, canned in syrup | 14 | 3 heaped tbsp | trace | trace | low | 55 |

| Food | Carbo-hydrate g | Portion size | Fat g | Protein g | Fibre | kCalories per portion |
|---|---|---|---|---|---|---|
| Peaches, whole, poached in natural juice | 16 | 1 peach | trace | 1 | med | 80 |
| Peaches, whole, poached in syrup | 16 | 1 peach | trace | 1 | med | 101 |
| Peaches, whole, poached in wine | 17 | 1 peach | trace | 1 | med | 136 |
| **Peanut brittle** | 34 | 1 standard bar | 9 | 3 | med | 226 |
| **Peanut butter** | 2 | 1 level tbsp | 8 | 3 | high | 93 |
| **Peanut butter and chocolate spread** | 5 | 1 level tbsp | 7 | 2 | med | 89 |
| **Peanut cookies** | 13 | 1 cookie | 6 | 2 | high | 116 |
| **Peanut sauce** | 8 | 5 level tbsp | 18 | 8 | med | 220 |
| **Peanuts**, dry-roasted | 1 | 1 small handful | 7 | 4 | med | 88 |
| Peanuts, raw, shelled | 3 | 25 g/1 oz/¼ cup | 11 | 6 | med | 141 |
| Peanuts, roasted, salted | 1 | 1 small handful | 8 | 4 | med | 90 |
| Peanuts and raisins | 5 | 1 small handful | 5 | 3 | med | 70 |
| **Pear** | 11 | 1 fruit, unpeeled | trace | trace | high | 45 |
| **Pear and apple pure fruit juice** | 20 | 1 tumbler | 0 | 0 | 0 | 78 |
| **Pear condé** | 51 | 1 average serving | 15 | 4 | med | 356 |
| **Pear drops** | 4 | 1 sweet (candy) | 0 | 0 | 0 | 16 |
| **Pear melba** | 32 | 1 average serving | 5 | 2 | low | 179 |
| Pears, canned in natural juice | 17 | 2 halves | trace | trace | med | 70 |
| Pears, canned in syrup | 25 | 2 halves | trace | trace | med | 100 |
| Pears, dried | 12 | 1 piece | trace | trace | high | 47 |

| Food | Carbo-hydrate g | Portion size | Fat g | Protein g | Fibre | kCalories per portion |
|---|---|---|---|---|---|---|
| Pears, dried, stewed | 34 | 3 heaped tbsp | trace | 1 | high | 127 |
| Pears, dried, stewed with sugar | 37 | 3 heaped tbsp | trace | 1 | high | 140 |
| Pears, poached in wine | 7 | 1 pear | trace | 1 | med | 139 |
| **Pears with chocolate sauce** | 87 | 1 average serving | 2 | 3 | high | 348 |
| **Peas**, dried, soaked and boiled | 20 | 3 heaped tbsp | 1 | 7 | high | 109 |
| Peas, fresh, shelled | 11 | 3 heaped tbsp | 1 | 7 | high | 83 |
| Peas, fresh, shelled cooked | 10 | 3 heaped tbsp | 2 | 7 | high | 79 |
| Peas, frozen, cooked | 10 | 3 heaped tbsp | 1 | 6 | high | 69 |
| Peas, garden, canned, drained | 13 | 3 heaped tbsp | 1 | 5 | high | 80 |
| Peas, marrowfat, canned, drained | 17 | 3 heaped tbsp | 1 | 7 | high | 100 |
| Peas, marrowfat, soaked and cooked | 18 | 3 heaped tbsp | 1 | 6 | high | 82 |
| Peas, mushy, canned | 14 | 3 heaped tbsp | 1 | 6 | med | 81 |
| Peas, processed, canned, drained | 17 | 3 heaped tbsp | 1 | 7 | high | 99 |
| Peas, split, soaked and boiled | 20 | 3 heaped tbsp | 16 | 10 | high | 262 |
| Peas, sugar snap | 8 | 10 pods | 1 | 5 | high | 57 |
| Peas, sugar snap, steamed or boiled | 5 | 3 heaped tbsp | 1 | 5 | high | 52 |
| **Pease pudding** | 20 | 3 heaped tbsp | 1 | 7 | high | 109 |
| **Pecan nuts**, shelled | 2 | 25 g/1 oz/¼ cup | 20 | 3 | high | 196 |
| **Pecan pie** | 64 | 1 average slice | 27 | 6 | med | 502 |

| Food | Carbo-hydrate g | Portion size | Fat g | Protein g | Fibre | kCalories per portion |
|---|---|---|---|---|---|---|
| **Pecorino cheese** | trace | 1 small chunk | 8 | 10 | 0 | 113 |
| **Peking duck** with pancakes | 32 | 1 portion with 6 small pancakes | 42 | 39 | high | 665 |
| **Penne rigate** (pasta shapes), dried, boiled | 42 | 1 average serving | 1 | 7 | med | 198 |
| Penne rigate, fresh, boiled | 45 | 1 average serving | 2 | 9 | med | 235 |
| **Penguin** chocolate bars, all flavours | 17 | 1 standard bar | 7 | 1 | low | 135 (average) |
| **Peperami** | trace | 1 stick | 12 | 5 | low | 132 |
| **Peppermint cordial**, diluted | 10 | 1 tumbler | trace | 0 | 0 | 36 |
| **Peppermints** | 5 | 1 mint | 0 | 0 | 0 | 18 |
| **Peperoni** | trace | 1 med slice | 2 | 1 | 0 | 27 |
| **Peperoni pizza** | 28 | 1 large slice | 10 | 14 | low | 255 |
| **Pepper** (bell), green | 4 | 1 medium pepper | trace | 1 | med | 22 |
| Pepper, green, roasted | 4 | 1 medium pepper | 5 | 1 | med | 45 |
| Pepper, green, stewed | 4 | 1 medium pepper | 1 | 1 | med | 27 |
| Pepper, orange/yellow | 7 | 1 medium pepper | trace | 1 | med | 35 |
| Pepper, orange/yellow, roasted | 7 | 1 medium pepper | 5 | 1 | med | 58 |
| Pepper, orange/yellow, stewed | 7 | 1 medium pepper | 1 | 2 | med | 39 |
| Pepper, red | 10 | 1 medium pepper | 1 | 1 | med | 48 |
| Pepper, red, roasted | 10 | 1 medium pepper | 6 | 2 | med | 71 |
| Pepper, red, stewed | 10 | 1 medium pepper | 1 | 2 | med | 51 |

| Food | Carbo-hydrate g | Portion size | Fat g | Protein g | Fibre | kCalories per portion |
|---|---|---|---|---|---|---|
| Pepper, stuffed with meat | 27 | 1 medium pepper | 8 | 23 | med | 266 |
| Pepper, stuffed with rice | 36 | 1 medium pepper | 5 | 7 | high | 202 |
| Pepsi | 22 | 1 tumbler | 0 | 0 | 0 | 88 |
| Pepsi, diet | trace | 1 tumbler | 0 | trace | 0 | 0 |
| Pepsi max | trace | 1 tumbler | 0 | trace | 0 | 1 |
| Pernod | trace | 1 single measure | 0 | trace | 0 | 55 |
| Perry, sparkling | 0 | 1 wineglass | 2 | trace | 0 | 70 |
| Persimmon | 8 | 1 fruit | trace | trace | low | 32 |
| Pesto sauce | trace | 1 level tbsp | 7 | 1 | low | 64 |
| Petit pois, cooked | 17 | 3 heaped tbsp | 1 | 7 | high | 49 |
| Petit suisse cheese | 1 | 1 small pot | 1 | 3 | 0 | 23 |
| Petits fours | 3 | 1 sweet (candy) | 1 | trace | low | 23 |
| Petticoat tails shortbread | 7 | 1 segment | 3 | 1 | low | 64 |
| Pheasant, roast | 0 | ¼ bird | 24 | 81 | 0 | 536 |
| Pheasant à la normande | 3 | ¼ bird | 46 | 91 | 0 | 675 |
| Pheasant casserole | 20 | ¼ bird | 30 | 85 | low | 588 |
| Physalis | trace | 1 fruit | trace | trace | low | 3 |
| Piccalilli | 3 | 1 level tbsp | trace | trace | low | 13 |
| Pickle, sweet | 5 | 1 level tbsp | trace | trace | low | 20 |
| Pickle, tomato | 6 | 1 level tbsp | trace | trace | low | 24 |
| Pickled egg | trace | 1 egg | 6 | 7 | 0 | 84 |
| Pickled onion, large | 1 | 1 onion | trace | trace | low | 4 |
| Pickled onion, silverskin | trace | 1 onion | trace | trace | low | 2 |

| Food | Carbo-hydrate g | Portion size | Fat g | Protein g | Fibre | kCalories per portion |
|---|---|---|---|---|---|---|
| **Picnic** chocolate bar | 29 | 1 standard bar | 11 | 4 | med | 230 |
| **Pigeon**, roast | 0 | ½ large or 1 small bird | 18 | 37 | 0 | 303 |
| **Pigeon casserole** | 8 | ½ large or 1 small bird | 20 | 39 | low | 333 |
| **Pigeon pie** | 21 | 1 average serving | 28 | 40 | med | 470 |
| **Pike**, grilled (broiled) | 0 | 1 piece of fillet | 1 | 38 | 0 | 175 |
| **Pikelets** | 19 | 1 pikelet | trace | 3 | low | 91 |
| **Pilaff** | 45 | 1 average serving | 9 | 7 | med | 286 |
| **Pilau rice** | 46 | 1 average serving | 2 | 4 | med | 212 |
| **Pilchards**, in tomato sauce, canned | 3 | 2 pilchards | 7 | 26 | low | 177 |
| **Pimientos**, canned, drained | 8 | 1 med pimiento | 1 | 1 | low | 21 |
| **Pimms** | 11 | 1 tumbler | 0 | trace | 0 | 146 |
| **Pina colada** | 32 | 1 cocktail | 3 | 1 | low | 252 |
| **Pine nuts** | 1 | 25 g/1 oz/¼ cup | 17 | 3 | med | 172 |
| **Pineapple** | 10 | 1 medium slice | trace | trace | med | 41 |
| Pineapple, chunks, canned in natural juice | 12 | 3 heaped tbsp | trace | trace | low | 47 |
| Pineapple, glacé (candied) | 4 | 1 piece | trace | trace | low | 13 |
| Pineapple, with kirsch | 29 | 2 medium slices | trace | trace | med | 132 |
| **Pineapple and grapefruit drink**, sparkling | 24 | 1 tumbler | trace | trace | 0 | 88 |

| Food | Carbo-hydrate g | Portion size | Fat g | Protein g | Fibre | kCalories per portion |
|---|---|---|---|---|---|---|
| **Pineapple and grapefruit pure fruit juice** | 24 | 1 tumbler | 0 | 0 | low | 94 |
| **Pineapple and grapefruit squash**, diluted | 22 | 1 tumbler | trace | trace | 0 | 96 |
| Pineapple and grapefruit squash, low-calorie, diluted | 5 | 1 tumbler | trace | 0 | 0 | 24 |
| **Pineapple flambé** | 24 | 1 med slice | 1 | 2 | med | 122 |
| **Pineapple pure fruit juice** | 21 | 1 tumbler | trace | 1 | low | 82 |
| **Pineapple sorbet** | 17 | 1 scoop | trace | trace | 0 | 65 |
| **Pineapple upside-down pudding** | 58 | 1 average serving | 14 | 4 | med | 367 |
| **Pineapple water ice** | 17 | 1 scoop | trace | trace | 0 | 65 |
| **Pink champagne** | 2 | 1 wineglass | 0 | trace | 0 | 114 |
| **Pink gin** | 0 | 1 cocktail | trace | trace | 0 | 56 |
| **Pink grapefruit** | 12 | 1 fruit | trace | 2 | med | 48 |
| Pink grapefruit, with sugar | 16 | ½ fruit | trace | 1 | med | 64 |
| Pink grapefruit, with sugar, grilled (broiled) | 16 | ½ fruit | trace | 1 | med | 64 |
| **Pinto beans**, refried | 15 | 3 heaped tbsp | 1 | 6 | high | 107 |
| Pinto beans, soaked and boiled | 24 | 3 heaped tbsp | 1 | 9 | high | 137 |
| **Piperade** | 18 | 1 average serving | 17 | 10 | med | 260 |
| **Pistachio nut ice cream** | 12 | 1 scoop | 4 | 2 | low | 91 |

| Food | Carbo-hydrate g | Portion size | Fat g | Protein g | Fibre | kCalories per portion |
|---|---|---|---|---|---|---|
| **Pistachio nuts**, unshelled | 1 | 1 small handful | 4 | 1 | high | 50 |
| **Pitta bread**, party size | 4 | 1 tiny bread | trace | 1 | low | 16 |
| Pitta bread, white | 36 | 1 bread | trace | 6 | med | 160 |
| Pitta bread, white, small | 18 | 1 small bread | trace | 3 | low | 80 |
| Pitta bread, wholemeal | 27 | 1 bread | 1 | 4 | high | 137 |
| **Pizza, cheese and tomato**, deep-pan | 30 | 1 large slice | 14 | 15 | med | 300 |
| Pizza, cheese and tomato, thin-crust *See also other flavours, e.g.* Ham and mushroom pizza | 25 | 1 large slice | 12 | 9 | med | 235 |
| **Plaice**, grilled (broiled) | 0 | 1 medium fish | 7 | 23 | 0 | 202 |
| Plaice, fillet, fried (sautéed), in batter | 24 | 1 fillet | 31 | 28 | low | 488 |
| Plaice, fillet, fried (sautéed), in breadcrumbs, | 15 | 1 fillet | 24 | 31 | low | 399 |
| Plaice, fillet, steamed or poached | 0 | 1 fillet | 3 | 33 | 0 | 162 |
| **Plantain**, boiled or steamed | 28 | ½ plantain | trace | 1 | med | 112 |
| Plantain, fried (sautéed) | 47 | ½ plantain | 9 | 1 | med | 267 |
| **Ploughman's lunch** | 54 | 1 average serving | 36 | 22 | med | 650 |
| **Plum**, large | 7 | 1 fruit | trace | trace | med | 30 |

| Food | Carbo-hydrate g | Portion size | Fat g | Protein g | Fibre | kCalories per portion |
|---|---|---|---|---|---|---|
| Plum, small | 2 | 1 fruit | trace | trace | med | 11 |
| Plum crumble | 51 | 1 average serving | 10 | 3 | med | 298 |
| Plum fool | 36 | 1 average serving | 8 | 5 | med | 227 |
| Plum jam (conserve) | 10 | 1 level tbsp | 0 | 0 | low | 39 |
| Plum pie | 14 | 1 average slice | 39 | 3 | med | 290 |
| Plum pudding | 49 | 1 average serving | 10 | 5 | med | 291 |
| Plum sauce, oriental | 6 | 1 level tbsp | trace | trace | low | 27 |
| Plums, canned in syrup | 15 | 3 heaped tbsp | trace | trace | low | 59 |
| Plums, stewed | 6 | 3 heaped tbsp | trace | 1 | med | 27 |
| Plums, stewed with sugar | 19 | 3 heaped tbsp | trace | 1 | med | 107 |
| Poires belle hélène | 87 | 1 average serving | 2 | 3 | high | 348 |
| Polenta (cornmeal) | 46 | 1 average serving | 1 | 5 | low | 214 |
| Polenta, with cheese | 46 | 1 average serving | 14 | 9 | low | 320 |
| Polenta, with meat sauce | 51 | 1 average serving | 18 | 17 | low | 431 |
| Pollack, baked | 0 | 1 piece of fillet | 2 | 38 | 0 | 178 |
| Polish pork sausage | 1 | ¼ ring | 16 | 8 | 0 | 185 |
| Polo mints | 34 | 1 tube | trace | 0 | 0 | 120 |
| Polo mints, sugar-free | 33 | 1 tube | 0 | 0 | 0 | 80 |
| Polony | 3 | 1 medium slice | 5 | 2 | 0 | 70 |
| Pomegranate | 12 | 1 fruit | trace | trace | high | 51 |
| Pommes dauphinoise | 12 | 1 average serving | 15 | 14 | med | 235 |

| Food | Carbo-hydrate g | Portion size | Fat g | Protein g | Fibre | kCalories per portion |
|------|------|------|------|------|------|------|
| **Pompano**, grilled (broiled) | 0 | 1 piece of fillet | 11 | 21 | 0 | 186 |
| **Pont l'évêque cheese** | trace | 1 small wedge | 8 | 6 | 0 | 101 |
| **Pontefract cakes** | 2 | 1 sweet (candy) | 0 | 0 | 0 | 8 |
| **Pop tarts**, all flavours | 36 | 1 tart | 6 | 3 | med | 202 (average) |
| **Poppadoms**, fried (sautéed) | 6 | 1 poppadom | 2 | 3 | low | 48 |
| Poppadoms, grilled (broiled) | 6 | 1 poppadom | trace | 3 | low | 35 |
| **Popcorn** | 25 | 1 small handful | 4 | trace | low | 137 |
| **Popcorn**, buttered | 12 | 1 small handful | 3 | trace | low | 72 |
| **Pork**, chop, barbecued | 1 | 1 chop | 9 | 28 | 0 | 210 |
| Pork, chop, lean, fried (sautéed) | 0 | 1 chop | 14 | 28 | 0 | 222 |
| Pork, chop, lean, grilled (broiled) | 0 | 1 chop | 9 | 28 | 0 | 199 |
| Pork, escalope, fried (sautéed) | 0 | 1 escalope | 7 | 31 | 0 | 185 |
| Pork, loin, smoked | 0 | 1 medium slice | 3 | 8 | 0 | 56 |
| Pork, minced (ground), lean, stewed | 0 | 1 average serving | 7 | 21 | 0 | 147 |
| Pork, roast, with crackling | 0 | 2 thick slices | 20 | 27 | 0 | 286 |
| Pork, roast, without crackling | 0 | 2 thick slices | 7 | 31 | 0 | 185 |
| **Pork, sweet and sour** | 31 | 1 average serving | 9 | 26 | med | 303 |

| Food | Carbo-hydrate g | Portion size | Fat g | Protein g | Fibre | kCalories per portion |
|---|---|---|---|---|---|---|
| **Pork and beef sausages**, thick, fried (sautéed) | 5 | 1 sausage | 8 | 5 | low | 115 |
| Pork and beef sausages, thick, grilled (broiled) | 5 | 1 sausage | 8 | 6 | low | 111 |
| Pork and beef sausages, thin, fried | 2 | 1 sausage | 4 | 2 | low | 57 |
| Pork and beef sausages, thin, grilled | 2 | 1 sausage | 4 | 3 | low | 55 |
| **Pork and vegetable stir-fry** | 18 | 1 average serving | 10 | 25 | high | 273 |
| **Pork belly**, grilled (broiled) | 0 | 1 medium slice | 35 | 21 | 0 | 398 |
| Pork belly, pickled | 0 | 1 medium slice | 22 | 20 | 0 | 280 |
| **Pork chop suey** | 34 | 1 average serving | 9 | 23 | med | 321 |
| **Pork chow mein** | 34 | 1 average serving | 8 | 29 | high | 323 |
| **Pork crackling** | 0 | 1 finger-sized piece | 13 | trace | 0 | 101 |
| **Pork kebab**, marinated and grilled (broiled) | 12 | 1 kebab | 10 | 22 | 0 | 227 |
| **Pork pie** | 45 | 1 individual pie | 49 | 18 | med | 677 |
| **Pork rillettes** | 0 | 2 level tbsp | 10 | 5 | 0 | 115 |
| **Pork sausages**, extra-lean, fried (sautéed) | 4 | 1 sausage | 5 | 6 | low | 92 |
| Pork sausages, extra-lean, grilled (broiled) | 4 | 1 sausage | 5 | 6 | low | 84 |

| Food | Carbo-hydrate g | Portion size | Fat g | Protein g | Fibre | kCalories per portion |
|---|---|---|---|---|---|---|
| Pork sausages, thick, fried | 4 | 1 sausage | 10 | 5 | low | 123 |
| Pork sausages, thick, grilled | 5 | 1 sausage | 10 | 7 | low | 117 |
| Pork sausages, thin, fried | 2 | 1 sausage | 5 | 3 | low | 61 |
| Pork sausages, thin, grilled | 2 | 1 sausage | 5 | 3 | low | 58 |
| **Pork spare ribs,** barbecued American-style | 2 | 2 medium ribs | 16 | 25 | 0 | 288 |
| Pork spare ribs, Chinese-style | 13 | 2 medium ribs | 17 | 25 | low | 310 |
| **Pork teriyaki** | 2 | 1 average serving | 5 | 18 | low | 133 |
| **Porridge,** instant *See* Ready brek | | | | | | |
| Porridge, made with semi-skimmed milk | 35 | 1 average serving | 6 | 9 | med | 217 |
| Porridge, made with skimmed milk | 35 | 1 average serving | 4 | 9 | med | 201 |
| Porridge, made with water | 29 | 1 average serving | 4 | 5 | med | 160 |
| **Port salut cheese** | trace | 1 small wedge | 8 | 7 | 0 | 100 |
| **Port,** ruby, tawny or white | 6 | 1 double measure | 0 | trace | 0 | 78 |
| **Pot au chocolat** | 19 | 1 individual pot | 5 | 2 | low | 136 |
| Pot au chocolat, with cream | 20 | 1 individual pot | 19 | 2 | low | 270 |
| **Pot noodle,** all flavours | 42 | 1 pot | 10 | 9 | low | 305 (average) |

| Food | Carbo-hydrate g | Portion size | Fat g | Protein g | Fibre | kCalories per portion |
|---|---|---|---|---|---|---|
| **Potato**, baked in jacket | **64** | 1 large potato | trace | 8 | high | 272 |
| Potato, baked in jacket, with butter | **64** | 1 large potato | 8 | 8 | high | 346 |
| **Potato cake** | **16** | 1 cake | 5 | 2 | low | 126 |
| **Potato chips** *See* Crisps | | | | | | |
| **Potato hoops**, all flavours | **14** | 1 small packet | 8 | 1 | low | 131 (average) |
| **Potato pancake** | **22** | 1 pancake | 11 | 5 | med | 207 |
| **Potato salad**, canned | **15** | 3 heaped tbsp | 10 | 2 | low | 176 |
| Potato salad, with French dressing | **27** | 3 heaped tbsp | 11 | 3 | med | 217 |
| Potato salad, with mayonnaise, home-made | **17** | 3 heaped tbsp | 12 | 3 | med | 200 |
| **Potato waffle**, cooked | **13** | 1 waffle | 3 | 1 | low | 84 |
| **Potato wedges** | **34** | 6 wedges | 4 | 10 | high | 205 |
| **Potatoes**, chipped (fries), home-made | **50** | 1 average serving | 11 | 6 | high | 312 |
| Potatoes, creamed | **15** | 1 average serving | 4 | 2 | med | 104 |
| Potatoes, croquette, shallow-fried | **11** | 1 croquette | 6 | 2 | med | 107 |
| Potatoes, duchesse | **8** | 1 piece | 2 | 2 | med | 82 |
| Potatoes, mashed, instant | **13** | 3 heaped tbsp | trace | 1 | low | 57 |
| Potatoes, mashed, with butter or margarine | **15** | 3 heaped tbsp | 4 | 2 | med | 104 |

| Food | Carbo-hydrate g | Portion size | Fat g | Protein g | Fibre | kCalories per portion |
|---|---|---|---|---|---|---|
| Potatoes, new, boiled or steamed | 18 | 3 small potatoes | trace | 1 | med | 75 |
| Potatoes, new, canned | 15 | 3 small potatoes | trace | 1 | low | 63 |
| Potatoes, steamed | 17 | 2 medium pieces | trace | 2 | med | 72 |
| Potatoes, roast | 26 | 2 medium pieces | 4 | 3 | med | 149 |
| Potatoes, scalloped | 11 | 1 average serving | 4 | 3 | med | 86 |
| Potted cheese | 1 | 1 small pot | 23 | 12 | 0 | 267 |
| Potted prawns (shrimp) | 0 | 1 small pot | 32 | 16 | 0 | 358 |
| Potted shrimps | 0 | 1 small pot | 31 | 10 | 0 | 324 |
| Poussin (Cornish hen), roast, with skin | 0 | 1 bird | 47 | 57 | 0 | 668 |
| Poussin, roast, without skin | 0 | 1 bird | 8 | 51 | 0 | 295 |
| Poussin, spatchcocked, grilled (broiled) | 0 | 1 bird | 30 | 36 | 0 | 428 |
| Praline ice cream | 12 | 1 scoop | 4 | 2 | low | 91 |
| Prawn, king (jumbo shrimp), plain-cooked | 0 | 1 prawn | trace | 2 | 0 | 10 |
| Prawn and vegetable stir-fry | 30 | 1 average serving | 5 | 20 | med | 250 |
| Prawn and avocado sandwiches | 35 | 1 round | 30 | 11 | med | 454 |
| Prawn and lettuce sandwiches | 34 | 1 round | 18 | 10 | med | 347 |
| Prawn biryani | 75 | 1 average serving | 32 | 11 | med | 707 |

| Food | Carbo-hydrate g | Portion size | Fat g | Protein g | Fibre | kCalories per portion |
|---|---|---|---|---|---|---|
| **Prawn chop suey** | 34 | 1 average serving | 2 | 16 | med | 225 |
| **Prawn choux balls** | 2 | 1 ball | 8 | 3 | low | 79 |
| **Prawn chow mein** | 28 | 1 average serving | 1 | 5 | high | 262 |
| **Prawn cocktail** | 4 | 1 average serving | 9 | 12 | low | 160 |
| **Prawn crackers** | 10 | 1 small handful | 1 | trace | low | 44 |
| **Prawn curry** | 36 | 1 average serving | 5 | 8 | med | 220 |
| **Prawn fajitas** | 34 | 2 fajitas | 13 | 15 | high | 300 |
| **Prawn jalfrezi** | 54 | 1 average serving | 9 | 26 | high | 465 |
| **Prawn mayonnaise sandwiches** | 36 | 1 round | 27 | 10 | med | 513 |
| **Prawn risotto** | 84 | 1 average serving | 18 | 47 | low | 389 |
| **Prawn rogan josh** | 17 | 1 average serving | 27 | 34 | med | 562 |
| **Prawn salad** | 5 | 1 average serving | 2 | 26 | high | 137 |
| **Prawn salad,** dressed | 5 | 1 average serving | 13 | 26 | high | 240 |
| **Prawn toast** | 2 | 1 toast | 4 | 2 | low | 53 |
| **Prawns** (shrimp), canned, drained | 0 | ½ small can | 1 | 18 | 0 | 80 |
| Prawns, cooked, peeled | 0 | 2 level tbsp | 1 | 12 | 0 | 53 |
| Prawns in garlic butter | trace | 1 average serving | 24 | 12 | 0 | 284 |
| **Pretzel flipz** | 33 | 1 small bag | 9 | 4 | low | 235 |
| **Pretzels** | 4 | 1 small handful | trace | trace | low | 20 |
| **Prickly pear** | 10 | 1 fruit | trace | 1 | high | 42 |
| **Processed cheese slice** | trace | 1 slice | 5 | 4 | 0 | 65 |
| **Profiteroles with chocolate sauce** | 33 | 1 average serving | 24 | 6 | med | 373 |

| Food | Carbo-hydrate g | Portion size | Fat g | Protein g | Fibre | kCalories per portion |
|---|---|---|---|---|---|---|
| **Provolone cheese** | 1 | 1 small wedge | 7 | 7 | 0 | 99 |
| **Prune juice** | 36 | 1 tumbler | trace | 1 | low | 136 |
| **Prunes** | 3 | 1 prune | trace | trace | high | 11 |
| Prunes, canned in natural juice | 20 | 3 heaped tbsp | trace | 1 | high | 79 |
| Prunes, canned in syrup | 23 | 3 heaped tbsp | trace | 1 | high | 90 |
| **Ptarmigan**, roast | 0 | 1 small or ½ large | 8 | 38 | 0 | 216 |
| **Puffed wheat**, dry | 17 | 25 g/1 oz/½ cup | trace | 4 | med | 80 |
| Puffed wheat, with semi-skimmed milk | 33 | 5 heaped tbsp | 2 | 10 | med | 185 |
| Puffed wheat, with skimmed milk | 33 | 5 heaped tbsp | trace | 10 | med | 169 |
| **Pumpernickel** | 20 | 1 medium slice | trace | 3 | med | 93 |
| **Pumpkin**, canned | 8 | 3 heaped tbsp | trace | 1 | med | 34 |
| Pumpkin, steamed or boiled | 2 | 3 heaped tbsp | trace | 1 | med | 13 |
| **Pumpkin pie** | 41 | 1 average slice | 14 | 7 | low | 316 |
| **Pumpkin seeds** | 3 | 1 small handful | 7 | 4 | high | 81 |
| **Puri** | 43 | 1 piece | 25 | 7 | med | 328 |

| Food | Carbo-hydrate g | Portion size | Fat g | Protein g | Fibre | kCalories per portion |
|------|-----------------|--------------|-------|-----------|-------|-----------------------|
| **Quail**, roast | 0 | 1 bird | 6 | 37 | 0 | 205 |
| **Quail's eggs**, cooked | trace | 1 egg | 1 | 1 | 0 | 15 |
| **Quality street chocolates** | 5 | 1 sweet (candy) | 2 | trace | 0 | 37 |
| **Quark** | trace | 1 level tbsp | trace | 2 | 0 | 15 |
| **Quarterpounder with cheese** | 37 | 1 burger in a bun | 27 | 31 | high | 516 |
| **Quavers** | 9 | 1 small packet | 6 | trace | low | 96 |
| **Queen cakes** | 26 | 1 individual cake | 15 | 2 | low | 245 |
| **Queen of puddings** | 46 | 1 average serving | 13 | 11 | low | 341 |
| **Queen scallops**, poached or steamed | 0 | 4 scallops | trace | 2 | 0 | 12 |
| **Quenelles**, fish | 3 | 1 ball/roll | 7 | 5 | 0 | 90 |
| **Quesadillas** | 27 | 3 pieces | 9 | 12 | high | 225 |
| **Quiche anglaise** | 17 | 1 large slice | 31 | 19 | low | 387 |
| **Quiche lorraine** *See also individual flavours, e.g. Cheese and onion quiche* | 24 | 1 large slice | 32 | 23 | low | 476 |
| **Quince** | 4 | 1 fruit | trace | trace | low | 17 |
| **Quince jelly** (clear conserve) | 13 | 1 level tbsp | trace | trace | 0 | 55 |
| **Quinoa** | 17 | 25 g/1 oz/3 tbsp | 1 | 3 | med | 93 |
| **Quinoa porridge**, made with semi-skimmed milk | 34 | 3 heaped tbsp | 4 | 9 | med | 206 |

| Food | Carbo-hydrate g | Portion size | Fat g | Protein g | Fibre | kCalories per portion |
|---|---|---|---|---|---|---|
| Quinoa porridge, made with skimmed milk | 34 | 3 heaped tbsp | 2 | 9 | med | 190 |
| Quinoa porridge, made with water | 28 | 3 heaped tbsp | 2 | 5 | med | 149 |
| **Quorn**, chunks | 2 | 1 average serving | 3 | 10 | high | 74 |
| Quorn, fillets | 2 | 1 fillet | 1 | 7 | med | 44 |
| Quorn, fillets, in breadcrumbs | 13 | 1 fillet | 10 | 10 | high | 185 |
| Quorn, minced (ground) | 1 | 1 average serving | 3 | 13 | high | 79 |
| **Quorn, sweet and sour** | 29 | 1 average serving | 1 | 5 | med | 149 |
| **Quorn burger** | 6 | 1 burger | 5 | 13 | high | 117 |
| **Quorn cottage pie** | 32 | 1 average serving | 6 | 8 | med | 212 |
| **Quorn fajitas** | 45 | 2 fajitas | 7 | 14 | high | 303 |
| **Quorn sausages** | 5 | 1 sausage | 5 | 13 | high | 115 |
| **Quorn southern burgers** | 12 | 1 burger | 10 | 11 | high | 178 |
| **Quorn spaghetti bolognese** | 38 | 1 average serving | 6 | 23 | high | 292 |
| **Quorn tikka masala**, with rice | 74 | 1 average serving | 21 | 20 | high | 540 |

| Food | Carbo-hydrate g | Portion size | Fat g | Protein g | Fibre | kCalories per portion |
|---|---|---|---|---|---|---|
| **Rabbit and vegetable stew** | 35 | 1 average serving | 3 | 38 | high | 404 |
| **Radicchio** | 1 | ½ head | trace | trace | med | 6 |
| **Radish** | trace | 1 radish | trace | trace | low | 1 |
| Radish, winter | 2 | 1 radish | trace | 1 | low | 12 |
| **Rainbow trout**, grilled (broiled) | 0 | 1 medium fish | 10 | 34 | 0 | 240 |
| **Raisin bread** | 15 | 1 medium slice | 7 | 2 | low | 86 |
| **Raisin fudge** | 15 | 1 square | 2` | trace | low | 87 |
| **Raisin wheats**, dry | 17 | 25 g/1 oz/½ cup | trace | 2 | high | 80 |
| Raisin wheats, with semi-skimmed milk | 34 | 3 heaped tbsp | 3 | 8 | high | 185 |
| Raisin wheats, with skimmed milk | 34 | 3 heaped tbsp | 1 | 8 | high | 169 |
| **Raisins**, seedless | 10 | 1 small handful | trace | trace | high | 41 |
| Raisins, stoned (pitted) | 11 | 1 small handful | trace | trace | high | 41 |
| **Rambutans** | 2 | 1 fruit | trace | trace | low | 7 |
| Rambutans, canned in syrup | 21 | 3 heaped tbsp | trace | 1 | low | 82 |
| **Raspberries** | 5 | 3 heaped tbsp | trace | 1 | med | 25 |
| Raspberries, canned in natural juice | 17 | 3 heaped tbsp | trace | 1 | med | 71 |
| Raspberries, canned in syrup | 22 | 3 heaped tbsp | trace | 1 | med | 88 |
| Raspberries, stewed | 4 | 3 heaped tbsp | trace | trace | med | 20 |
| Raspberries, stewed with sugar | 11 | 3 heaped tbsp | trace | 1 | med | 48 |
| **Raspberry jam** (conserve) | 10 | 1 level tbsp | 0 | trace | 0 | 39 |

| Food | Carbo-hydrate g | Portion size | Fat g | Protein g | Fibre | kCalories per portion |
|---|---|---|---|---|---|---|
| **Raspberry milkshake**, made with granules *See also* Milkshake | 23 | 1 tumbler | 3 | 6 | low | 138 |
| **Raspberry mousse** | 18 | 1 average serving | 6 | 4 | low | 137 |
| **Raspberry pavlova** | 45 | 1 average serving | 14 | 5 | med | 320 |
| **Raspberry ripple ice cream** | 12 | 1 scoop | 4 | 4 | 0 | 96 |
| **Raspberry sauce** | 7 | 2 level tbsp | trace | trace | med | 28 |
| **Raspberry sorbet** | 19 | 1 scoop | trace | trace | low | 57 |
| **Raspberry soufflé** | 21 | 1 average serving | 41 | 6 | 0 | 315 |
| **Raspberry tart** | 24 | 1 average slice | 18 | 3 | low | 271 |
| **Ratafia biscuits** (cookies) | 4 | 1 biscuit | trace | trace | low | 21 |
| **Ratatouille** | 11 | 3 heaped tbsp | 15 | 2 | high | 191 |
| **Ravioli**, dried, boiled | 45 | 1 average serving | 6 | 9 | med | 291 |
| Ravioli, fresh, boiled | 32 | 1 average serving | 8 | 12 | med | 248 |
| Ravioli, in beef and tomato sauce, canned | 23 | ½ large can | 5 | 7 | med | 154 |
| Ravioli, in tomato sauce, canned | 20 | ½ large can | 4 | 6 | med | 140 |
| **Ray** *See* Skate | | | | | | |
| **Ready-to-roll icing** (frosting) | 23 | 25 g/1 oz | 0 | 0 | 0 | 96 |
| Ready brek, dry | 15 | 25 g/1 oz/½ cup | 2 | 3 | med | 89 |
| Ready brek, with semi-skimmed milk | 31 | 5 heaped tbsp | 6 | 9 | high | 210 |
| Ready brek, with skimmed milk | 31 | 5 heaped tbsp | 3 | 9 | high | 191 |

| Food | Carbo-hydrate g | Portion size | Fat g | Protein g | Fibre | kCalories per portion |
|---|---|---|---|---|---|---|
| Ready brek, chocolate, dry | **16** | 25 g/1 oz/½ cup | 2 | 2 | med | 90 |
| Ready brek, chocolate, with skimmed milk | **33** | 5 heaped tbsp | 3 | 9 | high | 199 |
| Ready brek, chocolate, with semi-skimmed milk | **33** | 5 heaped tbsp | 5 | 9 | high | 215 |
| **Real fruit winders**, all flavours | **11** | 1 roll | 1 | trace | low | 55 (average) |
| **Red beet** *See* Beetroot | | | | | | |
| **Red bull** | **11** | 1 can | 0 | 0 | 0 | 45 |
| **Red kidney beans**, canned, drained | **18** | 3 heaped tbsp | 1 | 7 | high | 100 |
| Red kidney beans, dried, soaked and cooked | **17** | 3 heaped tbsp | trace | 8 | high | 103 |
| **Red Leicester cheese** | **trace** | 1 small wedge | 8 | 6 | 0 | 101 |
| **Red salmon** *See* Salmon | | | | | | |
| **Red snapper**, baked, stuffed | **12** | 1 medium fish | 2 | 19 | low | 146 |
| Red snapper, grilled (broiled) | **0** | 1 med fish | 3 | 45 | 0 | 218 |
| **Red Windsor cheese** | **trace** | 1 small wedge | 8 | 6 | 0 | 100 |
| **Red wine sauce** | **9** | 5 level tbsp | 2 | 1 | 0 | 63 |
| **Redcurrant jelly** (clear conserve) | **13** | 1 level tbsp | trace | trace | 0 | 55 |

| Food | Carbo-hydrate g | Portion size | Fat g | Protein g | Fibre | kCalories per portion |
|------|-----------------|--------------|-------|-----------|-------|-----------------------|
| **Redcurrants** | 7 | 3 heaped tbsp | trace | 1 | high | 28 |
| Redcurrants, frosted | 7 | 1 small bunch | trace | 1 | high | 27 |
| **Refried beans** | 15 | 3 heaped tbsp | 1 | 6 | high | 107 |
| **Revels** | 23 | 1 small packet | 6 | 2 | 0 | 173 |
| **Rhubarb**, canned in syrup | 8 | 3 heaped tbsp | trace | trace | low | 31 |
| Rhubarb, stewed | 1 | 3 heaped tbsp | trace | 1 | med | 7 |
| Rhubarb, stewed with sugar | 11 | 3 heaped tbsp | trace | 1 | med | 48 |
| **Rhubarb crumble** | 51 | 1 average serving | 10 | 3 | med | 297 |
| **Rhubarb fool** | 38 | 1 average serving | 8 | 5 | med | 237 |
| **Rhubarb pie** | 14 | 1 average slice | 39 | 3 | med | 290 |
| **Rhubarb sauce** | 34 | 2 level tbsp | trace | 1 | med | 137 |
| **Ribena**, diluted | 27 | 1 tumbler | 0 | trace | 0 | 103 |
| **Rice**, long-grain, boiled | 56 | 1 average serving | 2 | 5 | low | 248 |
| Rice, brown, boiled | 58 | 1 average serving | 2 | 5 | med | 254 |
| Rice, fried (sautéed) *See also* Egg fried rice *and* Special fried rice | 45 | 1 average serving | 6 | 4 | med | 236 |
| Rice, savoury | 47 | 1 average serving | 6 | 5 | med | 256 |
| **Rice and peas** | 53 | 1 average serving | 3 | 6 | high | 247 |
| **Rice cakes** | 7 | 1 individual cake | trace | 1 | low | 35 |
| **Rice drink** | 20 | 1 tumbler | trace | trace | 0 | 100 |
| **Rice krispies**, dry | 21 | 25 g/1 oz/½ cup | trace | 1 | low | 92 |
| Rice krispies, with semi-skimmed milk | 40 | 5 heaped tbsp | 2 | 6 | low | 205 |

| Food | Carbo-hydrate g | Portion size | Fat g | Protein g | Fibre | kCalories per portion |
|---|---|---|---|---|---|---|
| Rice krispies, with skimmed milk | **40** | 5 heaped tbsp | trace | 6 | low | 189 |
| **Rice milk** | **30** | 300 ml/½ pt/ 1¼ cups | 1 | trace | 0 | 150 |
| **Rice noodles**, boiled | **57** | 1 average serving | trace | 2 | low | 251 |
| **Rice pudding**, canned | **43** | ½ large can | 15 | 4 | low | 323 |
| Rice pudding, canned, low-fat | **23** | ½ large can | 2 | 7 | low | 136 |
| Rice pudding, made with semi-skimmed milk | **29** | 1 average serving | 2 | 6 | low | 150 |
| Rice pudding, made with skimmed milk | **29** | 1 average serving | trace | 6 | low | 134 |
| **Rich tea biscuits** (cookies) | **6** | 1 biscuit | 1 | 1 | low | 39 |
| **Ricicles**, dry | **22** | 25 g/1 oz/½ cup | trace | 1 | low | 90 |
| Ricicles, with semi-skimmed milk | **15** | 5 heaped tbsp | 2 | 4 | low | 201 |
| Ricicles, with skimmed milk | **15** | 5 heaped tbsp | trace | 4 | low | 185 |
| **Ricotta cheese**, made with semi-skimmed milk | **trace** | 1 good spoonful | 2 | 2 | 0 | 38 |
| Ricotta cheese, whole milk | **trace** | 1 good spoonful | 4 | 2 | 0 | 42 |
| **Rigatoni** (pasta shapes), dried, boiled | **42** | 1 average serving | 1 | 7 | med | 198 |
| Rigatoni, fresh, boiled | **45** | 1 average serving | 2 | 9 | med | 235 |

| Food | Carbo-hydrate g | Portion size | Fat g | Protein g | Fibre | kCalories per portion |
|---|---|---|---|---|---|---|
| **Ripple** chocolate bar | 19 | 1 standard bar | 10 | 3 | 0 | 175 |
| **Risotto** *See also individual flavours, e.g.* Mushroom risotto | 52 | 1 average serving | 14 | 4 | low | 336 |
| Risotto, sprinkled with cheese | 52 | 1 average serving | 22 | 14 | low | 449 |
| **Risotto alla milanese** | 58 | 1 average serving | 18 | 7 | med | 403 |
| **Rissoles** | 8 | 1 rissole | 9 | 5 | low | 134 |
| **Ritz original crackers** | 1 | 1 cracker | 1 | trace | low | 17 |
| Ritz cheese crackers | 1 | 1 cracker | 1 | trace | low | 17 |
| Ritz cheese sandwich crackers | 5 | 1 cracker | 2 | 1 | low | 45 |
| **Riva** chocolate bar | 14 | 1 standard bar | 8 | 2 | low | 136 |
| **Roasted nut** cereal bar | 24 | 1 bar | 8 | 3 | med | 181 |
| **Rock cakes** | 27 | 1 individual cake | 7 | 3 | low | 176 |
| **Rock salmon**, fried (sautéeed), in batter | 21 | 1 medium fillet | 44 | 30 | low | 580 |
| **Rocket** | trace | 1 good handful | trace | trace | med | 2 |
| **Rocky chocolate bars,** all flavours | 15 | 1 standard bar | 7 | 2 | low | 125 (average) |
| **Roes** *See* Cod roes *and* Herring roes | | | | | | |
| **Rollmop herring** | 6 | 1 roll | 12 | 12 | 0 | 180 |
| **Rolos** | 38 | 1 tube | 12 | 2 | 0 | 269 |
| **Romano cheese** | 1 | 1 small wedge | 8 | 9 | 0 | 110 |

| Food | Carbo-hydrate g | Portion size | Fat g | Protein g | Fibre | kCalories per portion |
|---|---|---|---|---|---|---|
| **Root beer** | 35 | 1 tumbler | 0 | 0 | 0 | 135 |
| **Roquefort cheese** | trace | 1 small wedge | 9 | 6 | 0 | 105 |
| **Rose hip syrup**, undiluted | 9 | 1 tbsp | 0 | trace | 0 | 35 |
| **Roses chocolates** | 5 | 1 sweet (candy) | 2 | trace | 0 | 39 |
| **Rosti** | 25 | 1 average serving | 5 | 3 | med | 156 |
| **Rotelli** (pasta shapes), dried, boiled | 42 | 1 average serving | 1 | 7 | med | 198 |
| Rotelli, fresh, boiled | 45 | 1 average serving | 2 | 9 | med | 235 |
| **Rouille** | 2 | 1 level tbsp | 15 | 1 | low | 151 |
| **Roulade** See *individual flavours, e.g.* Chocolate roulade | | | | | | |
| **Roulé**, garlic and herb cheese | 1 | 1 good spoonful | 7 | 2 | low | 77 |
| Roulé, light | 1 | 1 good spoonful | 2 | 2 | 0 | 28 |
| **Royal game soup** | 10 | 2 ladlefuls | 4 | 5 | low | 88 |
| **Royal icing** (frosting) | 15 | 1 level tbsp | 0 | trace | 0 | 58 |
| **Rum**, dark | trace | 1 single measure | 0 | trace | 0 | 55 |
| Rum, white | trace | 1 single measure | 0 | trace | 0 | 55 |
| Rum and black | 18 | 1 single measure | 0 | trace | 0 | 123 |
| Rum and coke | 6 | 1 single measure plus 1 mixer | 0 | trace | 0 | 94 |
| Rum and low-calorie cola | trace | 1 single measure plus 1 mixer | 0 | trace | 0 | 56 |
| **Rum and raisin fudge** | 15 | 1 square | 2 | trace | 0 | 87 |

| Food | Carbo-hydrate g | Portion size | Fat g | Protein g | Fibre | kCalories per portion |
|---|---|---|---|---|---|---|
| **Rum and raisin ice cream** | 12 | 1 scoop | 4 | 2 | low | 124 |
| **Rum and raisin sauce** | 32 | 2 level tbsp | 2 | 1 | low | 145 |
| **Rum baba** | 47 | 1 individual cake | 10 | 4 | low | 326 |
| **Rum butter** | 8 | 1 tbsp | 4 | trace | 0 | 73 |
| **Rum punch** | 15 | 1 wine glass | trace | trace | 0 | 116 |
| Rum sauce, made with semi-skimmed milk | 5 | 5 level tbsp | 2 | 1 | low | 50 |
| Rum sauce, made with skimmed milk | 5 | 5 level tbsp | trace | 1 | low | 47 |
| **Rump steak** See Steak, rump *or* sirloin | | | | | | |
| **Runner beans**, steamed or boiled | 2 | 3 heaped tbsp | trace | 1 | med | 18 |
| **Ruote** (pasta shapes), dried, boiled | 42 | 1 average serving | 1 | 7 | med | 198 |
| Ruote, fresh, boiled | 45 | 1 average serving | 2 | 9 | med | 235 |
| **Russian salad** | 5 | 2 good tbsp | 4 | 2 | high | 62 |
| **Rutabaga** See Swede | | | | | | |
| **Rye bread** | 11 | 1 medium slice | trace | 2 | med | 55 |
| Rye bread, light | 12 | 1 medium slice | trace | 2 | med | 35 |
| **Ryvita** | 5 | 1 crispbread | trace | 1 | med | 27 |

| Food | Carbo-hydrate g | Portion size | Fat g | Protein g | Fibre | kCalories per portion |
|---|---|---|---|---|---|---|
| **Sabayon sauce** | 4 | 5 level tbsp | 1 | 1 | 0 | 43 |
| **Sag aloo** | 21 | 1 average serving | 9 | 5 | high | 163 |
| **Sage Derby cheese** | trace | 1 small wedge | 9 | 6 | 0 | 101 |
| **Sago pudding,** canned | 27 | ½ large can | 7 | 4 | low | 167 |
| Sago pudding, made with semi-skimmed milk | 29 | 1 average serving | 2 | 6 | low | 150 |
| Sago pudding, made with skimmed milk | 29 | 1 average serving | trace | 6 | low | 134 |
| **Saint Paulin cheese** | trace | 1 small wedge | 8 | 7 | 0 | 100 |
| **Saithe** *See* Coley | | | | | | |
| **Salad cream** | 2 | 1 level tbsp | 5 | trace | 0 | 52 |
| Salad cream, reduced-calorie | 1 | 1 level tbsp | 2 | trace | 0 | 29 |
| **Salade niçoise** | 34 | 1 average serving | 11 | 21 | high | 308 |
| **Salami**, hard-cured | trace | 1 medium slice | 3 | 2 | 0 | 41 |
| Salami, moist-cured | trace | 1 medium slice | 5 | 3 | 0 | 57 |
| **Salmon**, baked, stuffed | 5 | 1 medium steak | 8 | 26 | low | 199 |
| Salmon, canned, drained | 0 | ½ small can | 4 | 10 | 0 | 155 |
| Salmon, grilled (broiled) | 0 | 1 piece of fillet | 25 | 39 | 0 | 367 |
| Salmon, in filo pastry (paste) | 8 | 1 portion | 17 | 42 | low | 495 |
| Salmon, poached or steamed | 0 | 1 piece of fillet | 23 | 35 | 0 | 345 |

| Food | Carbo-hydrate g | Portion size | Fat g | Protein g | Fibre | kCalories per portion |
|---|---|---|---|---|---|---|
| Salmon, smoked *See also entries for* Smoked salmon | 0 | 2 thin slices | 4 | 21 | 0 | 119 |
| Salmon, with hollandaise sauce | trace | 1 average serving | 48 | 43 | 0 | 559 |
| **Salmon and cucumber sandwiches** | 35 | 1 round | 21 | 14 | med | 378 |
| **Salmon en croûte** | 46 | 1 medium slice | 54 | 26 | low | 757 |
| **Salmon fish cakes,** fried (sautéed) | 15 | 1 cake | 11 | 8 | low | 213 |
| Salmon fish cakes, grilled (broiled) | 17 | 1 cake | 7 | 10 | low | 192 |
| **Salmon mousse** | 6 | 1 average serving | 6 | 9 | low | 205 |
| **Salmon paste** | trace | 1 level tbsp | 2 | 2 | 0 | 33 |
| **Salmon pâté** | 0 | 1 average serving | 28 | 12 | 0 | 308 |
| **Salmon quiche** | 17 | 1 large slice | 25 | 17 | low | 363 |
| **Salmon salad** | 5 | 1 average serving | 24 | 37 | high | 376 |
| Salmon salad, with mayonnaise | 5 | 1 average serving | 47 | 37 | high | 582 |
| **Salmon sandwiches** | 34 | 1 round | 21 | 14 | med | 374 |
| **Salsa**, fresh chilli | 4 | 1 level tbsp | trace | trace | med | 18 |
| Salsa, fresh tomato | 1 | 1 level tbsp | 1 | trace | med | 14 |
| **Salsify**, steamed or boiled | 9 | 3 heaped tbsp | trace | 1 | high | 23 |
| **Saltwater crayfish** *See* Dublin Bay prawns | | | | | | |
| **Sambals** | 4 | 2 level tbsp | 1 | 1 | med | 20 |
| **Samosa**, meat | 9 | 1 samosa | 28 | 2 | low | 300 |

| Food | Carbo-hydrate g | Portion size | Fat g | Protein g | Fibre | kCalories per portion |
|---|---|---|---|---|---|---|
| **Samosa, vegetable** | 11 | 1 samosa | 21 | 1 | med | 236 |
| **Sangria** | 4 | 1 wine glass | 0 | trace | 0 | 66 |
| **Sardine and tomato paste** | trace | 1 level tbsp | 1 | 3 | 0 | 23 |
| **Sardine pâté** | 0 | 1 average serving | 24 | 6 | 0 | 238 |
| **Sardines**, canned in oil, drained | 0 | ½ small can | 7 | 12 | 0 | 108 |
| Sardines, canned in tomato sauce | trace | ½ small can | 6 | 9 | low | 88 |
| Sardines, canned, on toast with butter | 8 | 3 sardines plus 1 slice of toast | 15 | 15 | low | 263 |
| Sardines, fresh, grilled (broiled) | 0 | 1 good-sized fish | 4 | 7 | 0 | 67 |
| **Satsuma** | 5 | 1 fruit | trace | trace | med | 23 |
| **Sauerkraut**, drained | 4 | 3 heaped tbsp | trace | 1 | med | 19 |
| **Sausage and bacon rolls** | 1 | 1 roll | 24 | 12 | low | 105 |
| **Sausage and egg mcmuffin** | 25 | 1 portion | 26 | 23 | med | 427 |
| **Sausage in batter**, fried (sautéed) | 23 | 1 sausage | 15 | 7 | low | 235 |
| **Sausage mcmuffin** | 26 | 1 portion | 23 | 13 | med | 360 |
| **Sausage roll**, cocktail | 3 | 1 small roll | 1 | 1 | low | 52 |
| Sausage roll, jumbo | 22 | 1 large roll | 24 | 4 | med | 477 |
| Sausage roll, puff pastry (paste) | 16 | 1 standard roll | 18 | 3 | low | 238 |
| Sausage roll, shortcrust pastry (basic pie crust) | 18 | 1 standard roll | 16 | 4 | low | 229 |

| Food | Carbo-hydrate g | Portion size | Fat g | Protein g | Fibre | kCalories per portion |
|---|---|---|---|---|---|---|
| **Sausages** See individual meats, e.g. Pork sausages | | | | | | |
| **Savarin** | 47 | 1 average slice | 10 | 4 | low | 326 |
| **Saveloy** | 6 | 1 sausage | 13 | 6 | low | 170 |
| **Savoury rice**, cooked | 24 | 1 average serving | 0 | 3 | med | 109 |
| **Scallion** See Spring onion | | | | | | |
| **Scallops**, fried (sautéed), in breadcrumbs | 1 | 1 scallop | 1 | 5 | low | 32 |
| Scallops, steamed or poached | 0 | 1 scallop | trace | 2 | 0 | 12 |
| **Scallops mornay** | 18 | 1 average serving | 3 | 27 | low | 210 |
| **Scaloppine**, fried (sautéed), in breadcrumbs | 20 | 1 scallopine | 15 | 32 | low | 335 |
| **Scampi**, fried (sautéed), in batter | 24 | 8 pieces | 16 | 16 | low | 360 |
| Scampi, fried (sautéed), in breadcrumbs | 29 | 8 pieces | 17 | 12 | low | 316 |
| **Scampi provençal** | 9 | 1 average serving | 10 | 25 | med | 286 |
| **Schloer** | 16 | 1 tumbler | 0 | trace | 0 | 61 |
| **Schnapps** | trace | 1 single measure | 0 | trace | 0 | 55 |
| **Schnitzel**, fried (sautéed), in breadcrumbs | 20 | 1 schnitzel | 15 | 32 | low | 335 |
| **Scone** (biscuit) | 27 | 1 scone | 7 | 4 | low | 181 |
| Scone, cheese | 21 | 1 scone | 9 | 5 | low | 175 |

| Food | Carbo-hydrate g | Portion size | Fat g | Protein g | Fibre | kCalories per portion |
|---|---|---|---|---|---|---|
| Scone, drop (small pancake) | 6 | 1 pancake | 2 | 1 | low | 44 |
| Scone, fruit | 26 | 1 scone | 5 | 4 | low | 158 |
| Scone, griddle | 6 | 1 scone | 2 | 1 | low | 44 |
| Scone, plain, with butter | 27 | 1 scone | 15 | 4 | low | 255 |
| Scone, plain, with low-fat spread | 27 | 1 scone | 11 | 5 | low | 220 |
| Scone, sweet | 32 | 1 scone | 7 | 4 | low | 201 |
| Scone, sweet, with butter | 32 | 1 scone | 15 | 4 | low | 275 |
| Scone, sweet, with low-fat spread | 32 | 1 scone | 11 | 5 | low | 240 |
| Scone, with clotted cream and jam (conserve) | 37 | 1 scone | 16 | 4 | low | 308 |
| Scotch broth, canned | 14 | 2 ladlefuls | 2 | 4 | med | 88 |
| Scotch broth, home-made | 19 | 2 ladlefuls | 3 | 12 | high | 156 |
| Scotch egg | 16 | 1 egg | 20 | 14 | low | 301 |
| Scotch pancake | 6 | 1 pancake | 2 | 1 | low | 44 |
| Scotch pie | 24 | 1 individual pie | 5 | 8 | med | 225 |
| Scotch woodcock | 18 | 1 med slice | 39 | 19 | low | 487 |
| Scrambled eggs, on toast with butter | 19 | 2 eggs plus 1 slice of toast | 37 | 16 | low | 463 |
| Sea bass, grilled (broiled) | 0 | 1 piece of fillet | 4 | 28 | 0 | 153 |
| Seafood cocktail | 4 | 1 cocktail | 9 | 6 | low | 134 |
| Seafood enchiladas | 78 | 2 enchiladas | 14 | 32 | med | 562 |

| Food | Carbo-hydrate g | Portion size | Fat g | Protein g | Fibre | kCalories per portion |
|---|---|---|---|---|---|---|
| Seafood lasagne | 32 | 1 average serving | 16 | 22 | high | 351 |
| Seafood pasta | 62 | 1 average serving | 4 | 40 | high | 460 |
| Seafood pasta salad | 29 | 1 average serving | 5 | 24 | med | 261 |
| Seafood pizza, thin-crust | 25 | 1 large slice | 13 | 12 | med | 250 |
| Seafood pizza, deep-pan | 30 | 1 large slice | 15 | 18 | med | 315 |
| Seafood salad | 5 | 1 average serving | 2 | 17 | high | 106 |
| Seafood salad, with mayonnaise | 5 | 1 average serving | 24 | 17 | high | 312 |
| Seafood sticks | 1 | 1 stick | trace | 2 | 0 | 12 |
| Seakale, steamed or boiled | 1 | 3 heaped tbsp | 1 | 2 | med | 24 |
| Seaweed | 1 | 2 good tbsp | trace | trace | low | 4 |
| Seaweed, deep-fried | 3 | 3 heaped tbsp | 12 | 12 | med | 131 |
| Seed cake | 58 | 1 average slice | 20 | 6 | low | 423 |
| Semolina (cream of wheat), canned | 27 | ½ large can | 5 | 3 | low | 172 |
| Semolina, made with semi-skimmed milk | 29 | 1 average serving | 2 | 6 | low | 150 |
| Semolina, made with skimmed milk | 29 | 1 average serving | trace | 6 | low | 134 |
| Sesame seeds | trace | 1 level tbsp | 9 | 3 | high | 90 |
| Seven-up | 22 | 1 tumbler | 0 | 0 | 0 | 88 |
| Seven-up, diet | 0 | 1 tumbler | 0 | 0 | 0 | 3 |
| Seviche | 3 | 1 average serving | 18 | 20 | low | 193 |
| Shandy | 13 | 1 tumbler | trace | trace | 0 | 48 |

| Food | Carbo-hydrate g | Portion size | Fat g | Protein g | Fibre | kCalories per portion |
|---|---|---|---|---|---|---|
| **Shark steak**, fried (sautéed) | 0 | 1 medium steak | 13 | 32 | 0 | 283 |
| Shark steak, grilled (broiled) | 0 | 1 medium steak | 8 | 32 | 0 | 260 |
| **Shark's fin soup** | 8 | 2 ladlefuls | 7 | 7 | 0 | 99 |
| **Sheep's milk** | 15 | 300 ml/½ pt/ 1¼ cups | 18 | 16 | 0 | 285 |
| **Shepherd's pie** | 25 | 1 average serving | 19 | 24 | med | 330 |
| **Sherbet dip** | 19 | 1 small packet | 0 | 0 | 0 | 78 |
| **Sherbet drink** | 20 | 1 tumbler | 1 | trace | 0 | 91 |
| **Sherbet fountain** | 21 | 1 tube | 0 | trace | 0 | 88 |
| **Sherbet lemons** | 5 | 1 sweet (candy) | 0 | 0 | 0 | 20 |
| **Sherbet oranges** | 5 | 1 sweet (candy) | 0 | 0 | 0 | 20 |
| **Sherbet pips** | 1 | 1 pip | 0 | 0 | 0 | 4 |
| **Sherried chicken** | 7 | ¼ small chicken | 4 | 29 | low | 197 |
| **Sherry**, dry (fino) | 1 | 1 double measure | 0 | trace | 0 | 58 |
| Sherry, medium (amontillado) | 2 | 1 double measure | 0 | trace | 0 | 59 |
| Sherry, sweet (oloroso) | 3 | 1 double measure | 0 | trace | 0 | 68 |
| **Shiitake mushrooms**, dried, reconstituted, stewed | 7 | 1 good tbsp | trace | 1 | low | 35 |
| Shiitake mushrooms, fresh, fried (sautéed) | 6 | 2 good tbsp | 5 | 1 | low | 50 |
| Shiitake mushrooms, fresh, stewed | 6 | 2 good tbsp | trace | 1 | low | 27 |
| **Shish kebabs** | 0 | 1 kebab | 8 | 25 | 0 | 176 |

| Food | Carbo-hydrate g | Portion size | Fat g | Protein g | Fibre | kCalories per portion |
|------|------|------|------|------|------|------|
| **Shortbread fingers** | 8 | 1 finger | 3 | 1 | low | 67 |
| **Shortcake biscuits** (cookies) | 6 | 1 biscuit | 2 | trace | low | 43 |
| **Shredded wheat**, dry | 15 | 1 biscuit | trace | 2 | high | 74 |
| Shredded wheat, with semi-skimmed milk | 36 | 2 biscuits | 2 | 9 | high | 205 |
| Shredded wheat, with skimmed milk | 36 | 2 biscuits | 1 | 9 | high | 189 |
| Shredded wheat bitesize, dry | 17 | 25 g/1 oz/½ cup | trace | 3 | high | 84 |
| Shredded wheat bitesize, with semi-skimmed milk | 37 | 3 heaped tbsp | 3 | 9 | high | 208 |
| Shredded wheat bitesize, with skimmed milk | 37 | 3 heaped tbsp | 1 | 9 | high | 192 |
| **Shreddies**, dry | 18 | 25 g/1 oz/½ cup | trace | 2 | high | 86 |
| Shreddies, with semi-skimmed milk | 38 | 5 heaped tbsp | 3 | 9 | high | 213 |
| Shreddies, with skimmed milk | 38 | 5 heaped tbsp | 1 | 9 | high | 197 |
| Shreddies, chocolate, dry | 20 | 25 g/1 oz/½ cup | trace | 2 | med | 91 |
| Shreddies, chocolate, with semi-skimmed milk | 42 | 5 heaped tbsp | 3 | 8 | high | 224 |
| Shreddies, chocolate, with skimmed milk | 42 | 5 heaped tbsp | 1 | 8 | high | 208 |

| Food | Carbo-hydrate g | Portion size | Fat g | Protein g | Fibre | kCalories per portion |
|------|------------------|--------------|-------|-----------|-------|------------------------|
| Shreddies, frosted, dry | 20 | 25 g/1 oz/½ cup | trace | 2 | high | 91 |
| Shreddies, frosted, with semi-skimmed milk | 43 | 5 heaped tbsp | 3 | 7 | high | 224 |
| Shreddies, frosted, with skimmed milk | 43 | 5 heaped tbsp | 1 | 7 | high | 208 |
| **Shrimp** See Prawns | | | | | | |
| Shrimps, canned, drained | 0 | ½ small can | trace | 18 | 0 | 80 |
| Shrimps, grey or pink, cooked, peeled | 0 | 2 level tbsp | trace | 8 | 0 | 15 |
| Shrimps, potted | 0 | 1 small pot | 32 | 16 | 0 | 358 |
| **Shropshire blue cheese** | trace | 1 small wedge | 7 | 5 | 0 | 87 |
| **Sieved tomatoes** See Passata | | | | | | |
| **Sild**, in oil, drained | 0 | ½ small can | 7 | 12 | 0 | 108 |
| **Silverskin onions** | trace | 1 onion | trace | trace | low | 2 |
| **Simnel cake** | 49 | 1 average slice | 11 | 4 | med | 298 |
| **Skate wings**, in batter | 9 | 1 medium wing | 22 | 33 | low | 367 |
| Skate wings, in black butter | trace | 1 med wing | 41 | 31 | 0 | 470 |
| **Skippers**, in oil, drained | 0 | ½ small can | 7 | 12 | 0 | 108 |
| **Skips** | 10 | 1 small packet | 5 | 1 | low | 87 |
| **Slivovitz** | trace | 1 single measure | 0 | trace | 0 | 55 |
| **Sloe gin** | 8 | 1 single measure | 0 | trace | 0 | 35 |

| Food | Carbo-hydrate g | Portion size | Fat g | Protein g | Fibre | kCalories per portion |
|------|-----------------|--------------|-------|-----------|-------|------------------------|
| **Smacks**, dry | 21 | 25 g/1 oz/½ cup | trace | 2 | low | 95 |
| Smacks, with semi-skimmed milk | **40** | 5 heaped tbsp | 3 | 7 | low | 209 |
| Smacks, with skimmed milk | **40** | 5 heaped tbsp | 1 | 7 | low | 193 |
| **Smarties** (M&Ms) | 26 | 1 tube | 9 | 2 | 0 | 170 |
| **Smelts**, fried (sautéed), in seasoned flour | 5 | 5 fish | 47 | 19 | low | 525 |
| **Smoked chicken breast** | trace | 1 medium slice | 1 | 2 | 0 | 23 |
| **Smoked fish** See individual fish, e.g. Salmon, smoked, also Smoked haddock and Smoked salmon | | | | | | |
| **Smoked haddock roulade** | 16 | 1 average serving | 20 | 30 | low | 377 |
| **Smoked pork ring** | 1 | ¼ ring | 16 | 8 | 0 | 185 |
| **Smoked salmon** | 0 | 2 thin slices | 4 | 21 | 0 | 119 |
| **Smoked salmon sandwiches** | 34 | 1 round | 19 | 15 | med | 363 |
| **Smoked salmon and cream cheese bagel** | 44 | 1 bagel | 12 | 17 | med | 353 |
| **Smoked salmon and cream cheese sandwiches** | 34 | 1 round | 26 | 15 | med | 429 |
| **Smoked salmon pâté** | 0 | 1 average serving | 26 | 10 | 0 | 273 |

| Food | Carbo-hydrate g | Portion size | Fat g | Protein g | Fibre | kCalories per portion |
|---|---|---|---|---|---|---|
| **Smoked turkey breast** | **trace** | 1 medium slice | trace | 4 | 0 | 21 |
| **Snack** shortcake | **5** | 1 biscuit (cookie) | 2 | trace | low | 40 |
| Snack wafer bar | **7** | 1 finger | 4 | trace | 0 | 65 |
| **Snails**, in garlic butter | **trace** | 6 snails | 25 | 12 | low | 311 |
| **Snapper**, grilled (broiled) | **0** | 1 medium fish | 3 | 45 | 0 | 218 |
| **Snickers** chocolate bar | **36** | 1 standard bar | 18 | 6 | low | 329 |
| Snickers ice cream bar | **20** | 1 standard bar | 15 | 4 | low | 230 |
| **Snow peas** *See* Mangetout | | | | | | |
| **Soba noodles**, cooked | **48** | 1 average serving | trace | 11 | high | 228 |
| **Soda bread**, brown | **15** | 1 thick slice | 2 | 2 | low | 80 |
| Soda bread, white | **12** | 1 thick slice | 2 | 2 | low | 82 |
| **Softgrain bread** *See* Bread | | | | | | |
| **Sole** *See individual varieties, and cooking methods, e.g.* Dover sole, Sole meunière, *etc.* | | | | | | |
| **Sole meunière** | **trace** | 1 medium fish | 22 | 44 | 0 | 376 |
| **Sole mornay** | **7** | 1 medium fillet | 12 | 47 | low | 243 |
| **Sole véronique** | **11** | 1 medium fillet | 6 | 41 | low | 184 |
| **Solero** ice lolly | **20** | 1 lolly | 4 | 2 | 0 | 130 |
| **Somen noodles**, boiled | **48** | 1 average serving | trace | 7 | med | 230 |

| Food | Carbo-hydrate g | Portion size | Fat g | Protein g | Fibre | kCalories per portion |
|---|---|---|---|---|---|---|
| **Soufflé** See *individual flavours,* e.g. Cheese soufflé | | | | | | |
| **Soufflé omelette,** savoury | trace | 2 eggs | 22 | 14 | 0 | 256 |
| Soufflé omelette, sweet | 10 | 2 eggs | 22 | 14 | 0 | 374 |
| **Soupe au pistou,** canned | 13 | 2 ladlefuls | 1 | 2 | med | 60 |
| **Soured (dairy sour) cream and chive dressing** | trace | 1 level tbsp | 3 | trace | low | 38 |
| **Soused herring** | 6 | 1 roll | 12 | 12 | 0 | 180 |
| **Soused mackerel** | 6 | 1 roll | 9 | 16 | 0 | 165 |
| **Southern comfort** | 4 | 1 single measure | 0 | trace | 0 | 70 |
| **Southern fried chicken** | 19 | 2 pieces | 29 | 36 | low | 494 |
| **Soy sauce** | 1 | 1 tsp | 0 | 1 | 0 | 10 |
| **Soya beans,** canned, drained | 5 | 3 heaped tbsp | 7 | 13 | high | 140 |
| Soya beans, dried, soaked and cooked | 5 | 3 heaped tbsp | 7 | 14 | high | 141 |
| **Soya cheese** | trace | 1 small wedge | 9 | 6 | 0 | 106 |
| **Soya cream substitute** | 1 | 1 level tbsp | 3 | trace | low | 28 |
| **Soya desserts**, all flavours | 19 | 1 individual pot | 2 | 3 | low | 103 (average) |
| **Soya ice desserts**, all flavours | 5 | 1 scoop | 2 | trace | low | 44 (average) |
| **Soya milk,** sweetened | 12 | 300 ml/½ pt/ 1¼ cups | 5 | 9 | low | 120 |

| Food | Carbo-hydrate g | Portion size | Fat g | Protein g | Fibre | kCalories per portion |
|---|---|---|---|---|---|---|
| Soya milk, unsweetened | 2 | 300 ml/½ pt/ 1¼ cups | 6 | 9 | low | 96 |
| **Soya yoghurt** | 5 | 1 individual pot | 5 | 6 | low | 90 |
| **Spaghetti**, dried, boiled | 51 | 1 average serving | 2 | 8 | med | 239 |
| Spaghetti, dried, wholemeal, boiled | 152 | 1 average serving | 6 | 31 | high | 259 |
| Spaghetti, fresh, boiled | 57 | 1 average serving | 2 | 11 | med | 301 |
| Spaghetti, with clams | 52 | 1 average serving | 6 | 36 | med | 433 |
| Spaghetti, with meatballs | 80 | 1 average serving | 31 | 36 | med | 718 |
| Spaghetti, with sausages in tomato sauce, canned | 25 | 1 small can | 9 | 8 | med | 116 |
| Spaghetti, with tomato sauce | 71 | 1 average serving | 13 | 12 | high | 432 |
| Spaghetti, with tomato sauce, canned | 27 | 1 small can | 1 | 4 | med | 128 |
| Spaghetti, with tomato sauce, no-added-sugar, canned | 20 | 1 small can | 1 | 4 | med | 101 |
| **Spaghetti alfredo** | 67 | 1 average serving | 13 | 23 | high | 478 |
| **Spaghetti bolognese** | 56 | 1 average serving | 19 | 20 | med | 456 |
| **Spaghetti carbonara** | 56 | 1 average serving | 22 | 10 | med | 402 |
| **Spaghetti hoops**, canned | 26 | 1 small can | 1 | 4 | med | 122 |

| Food | Carbo-hydrate g | Portion size | Fat g | Protein g | Fibre | kCalories per portion |
|------|-----------------|--------------|-------|-----------|-------|-----------------------|
| Spaghetti hoops with hot dogs, canned | 22 | 1 small can | 8 | 6 | low | 180 |
| **Spaghetti napoletana** | 71 | 1 average serving | 13 | 12 | high | 432 |
| **Spam** | trace | 1 slice | 8 | 4 | 0 | 86 |
| **Spanish omelette** | 17 | 2 eggs | 22 | 16 | med | 328 |
| **Spanish rice** | 46 | 1 average serving | 2 | 6 | high | 228 |
| **Spare ribs** *See* Pork spare ribs | | | | | | |
| **Special fried rice** | 54 | 1 average serving | 9 | 17 | high | 362 |
| **Special K**, dry | 18 | 25 g/1 oz/½ cup | trace | 4 | low | 92 |
| Special K, with semi-skimmed milk | 36 | 5 heaped tbsp | trace | 10 | low | 205 |
| Special K, with skimmed milk | 36 | 5 heaped tbsp | trace | 10 | low | 189 |
| Special K red berries, dry | 18 | 25 g/1 oz/½ cup | trace | 3 | low | 92 |
| Special K red berries, with semi-skimmed milk | 36 | 5 heaped tbsp | 2 | 10 | low | 205 |
| Special K red berries, with skimmed milk | 36 | 5 heaped tbsp | trace | 10 | low | 189 |
| **Spinach** | 1 | 1 good handful | trace | 1 | med | 12 |
| Spinach, cooked | 1 | 3 heaped tbsp | 1 | 2 | med | 19 |
| Spinach, frozen, cooked | trace | 3 heaped tbsp | 1 | 3 | med | 21 |
| **Spinach and bacon salad** | 9 | 1 average serving | 44 | 18 | med | 451 |
| **Spinach roulade** | 16 | 1 average serving | 20 | 21 | high | 327 |

| Food | Carbo-hydrate g | Portion size | Fat g | Protein g | Fibre | kCalories per portion |
|---|---|---|---|---|---|---|
| **Spinach soup**, home-made | 31 | 2 ladlefuls | trace | 4 | med | 132 |
| **Spirali** (pasta shapes), dried, boiled | 42 | 1 average serving | 1 | 7 | med | 198 |
| Spirali, fresh, boiled | 45 | 1 average serving | 2 | 9 | med | 235 |
| **Split ice lolly**, any flavour | 13 | 1 lolly | 3 | 1 | 0 | 83 |
| **Split pea soup**, canned | 24 | 1 average serving | 2 | 8 | high | 142 |
| **Sponge cake** | 26 | 1 average slice | 13 | 3 | low | 229 |
| Sponge cake, fatless | 26 | 1 average slice | 3 | 5 | low | 147 |
| Sponge cake, fatless, filled with cream | 36 | 1 average slice | 22 | 5 | low | 343 |
| Sponge cake, fatless, filled with jam (conserve) | 38 | 1 average slice | 3 | 5 | low | 181 |
| Sponge cake, Victoria, filled with cream | 52 | 1 average slice | 31 | 4 | low | 490 |
| Sponge cake, Victoria, filled with jam (conserve) | 64 | 1 average slice | 5 | 4 | low | 302 |
| **Sponge (lady) fingers** | 6 | 1 finger | 1 | 1 | low | 40 |
| **Sporties**, dry | 19 | 25 g/1 oz/½ cup | trace | 2 | high | 89 |
| Sporties, with semi-skimmed milk | 37 | 5 heaped tbsp | 3 | 8 | high | 203 |
| Sporties, with skimmed milk | 37 | 5 heaped tbsp | 1 | 8 | high | 187 |
| **Spotted dick** | 52 | 1 average serving | 16 | 7 | med | 350 |

| Food | Carbo-hydrate g | Portion size | Fat g | Protein g | Fibre | kCalories per portion |
|------|------|------|------|------|------|------|
| **Sprats**, fried (sautéed) | 4 | 5 fish | 35 | 14 | low | 393 |
| **Spring greens** (collard greens), steamed or boiled | 2 | 3 heaped tbsp | 1 | 2 | med | 20 |
| **Spring onions** (scallions) | trace | 1 medium onion | trace | trace | low | 3 |
| **Spring roll**, large | 21 | 1 large roll | 12 | 7 | low | 217 |
| Spring roll, small | 7 | 1 small roll | 3 | 3 | low | 70 |
| **Spring vegetable soup**, canned | 13 | 2 ladlefuls | trace | 2 | med | 62 |
| Spring vegetable soup, packet | 9 | 2 ladlefuls | 4 | 2 | low | 80 |
| **Sprite** | 22 | 1 tumbler | 0 | 0 | 0 | 85 |
| Sprite, diet | 0 | 1 tumbler | 0 | 0 | 0 | 5 |
| **Squab**, roast | 0 | 1 bird | 18 | 37 | 0 | 303 |
| **Squab pie** | 21 | 1 average serving | 28 | 40 | med | 470 |
| **Squash** See Marrow | | | | | | |
| Squash, butternut | 2 | ½ med squash | trace | trace | low | 9 |
| **Squash, fruit**, diluted See individual flavours, e.g. Orange squash | | | | | | |
| **Squid**, stewed in olive oil | 0 | 1 average serving | 31 | 13 | 0 | 336 |
| Squid, stuffed | 4 | 1 squid | 10 | 6 | low | 85 |
| Squid rings, fried (sautéed), in batter, | 19 | 1 average serving | 12 | 14 | low | 235 |
| **Squid risotto** | 52 | 1 average serving | 15 | 9 | low | 369 |
| **Starfruit** | 7 | 1 fruit | trace | trace | med | 30 |

| Food | Carbo-hydrate g | Portion size | Fat g | Protein g | Fibre | kCalories per portion |
|---|---|---|---|---|---|---|
| **Starburst sweets** (candies) | 38 | 1 tube | 3 | trace | 0 | 185 |
| **Start**, dry | 20 | 25 g/1 oz/½ cup | trace | 2 | med | 90 |
| Start, with semi-skimmed milk | 38 | 5 heaped tbsp | 3 | 7 | med | 201 |
| Start, with skimmed milk | 38 | 5 heaped tbsp | 1 | 7 | med | 185 |
| **Steak**, fillet, fried (sautéed) | 0 | 1 medium fillet | 21 | 48 | 0 | 359 |
| Steak, fillet, grilled (broiled) | 0 | 1 medium fillet | 16 | 48 | 0 | 336 |
| Steak, rump or sirloin, fried | 0 | 1 medium steak | 25 | 50 | 0 | 430 |
| Steak, rump or sirloin, grilled | 0 | 1 medium steak | 21 | 48 | 0 | 381 |
| **Steak and kidney pie** | 28 | 1 average serving | 32 | 26 | med | 500 |
| Steak and kidney pie, individual | 38 | 1 pie | 31 | 13 | med | 484 |
| **Steak and kidney pudding** | 24 | 1 average serving | 23 | 34 | low | 431 |
| **Steak and onions** | 8 | 1 medium steak | 27 | 49 | med | 463 |
| **Steak au poivre** | 1 | 1 medium steak | 29 | 48 | 0 | 455 |
| **Steak chasseur** | 7 | 1 medium steak | 21 | 49 | 0 | 417 |
| **Steak diane** | 3 | 1 medium steak | 28 | 51 | low | 488 |
| **Steak sandwiches** | 34 | 1 round | 38 | 53 | low | 685 |
| **Steamed sponge pudding** | 45 | 1 average serving | 16 | 6 | med | 340 |
| **Steamed suet pudding** | 34 | 1 average serving | 12 | 3 | low | 221 |

| Food | Carbo-hydrate g | Portion size | Fat g | Protein g | Fibre | kCalories per portion |
|---|---|---|---|---|---|---|
| **Stem lettuce** *See* Chinese leaves | | | | | | |
| **Sticky toffee pudding** | 47 | 1 average serving | 12 | 3 | low | 313 |
| **Stifado** | 45 | 1 average serving | 16 | 6 | med | 565 |
| **Stilton cheese**, blue | trace | 1 small wedge | 9 | 6 | 0 | 103 |
| Stilton cheese, white | trace | 1 small wedge | 8 | 6 | 0 | 94 |
| **Stock cube**, chicken | 3 | 1 cube | 2 | 1 | 0 | 32 |
| Stock cube, meat | 2 | 1 cube | 2 | 1 | 0 | 32 |
| Stock cube, vegetable | 3 | 1 cube | 2 | 1 | 0 | 33 |
| **Stollen** | 26 | 1 slice | 13 | 2 | med | 177 |
| **Stout** | 6 | 1 small | trace | 1 | 0 | 117 |
| **Straw mushrooms**, canned, drained | 1 | ¼ med can | trace | 1 | 0 | 7 |
| **Strawberries** | 6 | 3 heaped tbsp | trace | 1 | med | 27 |
| Strawberries, canned in natural juice | 13 | 3 heaped tbsp | trace | trace | med | 48 |
| Strawberries, canned in syrup | 17 | 3 heaped tbsp | trace | trace | med | 65 |
| **Strawberry cheesecake** | 32 | 1 average slice | 17 | 5 | low | 296 |
| **Strawberry dessert** | 16 | 1 small pot | 3 | 3 | 0 | 101 |
| **Strawberry ice cream** | 12 | 1 scoop | 4 | 1 | 0 | 89 |
| **Strawberry milkshake**, made with granules and semi-skimmed milk | 23 | 1 tumbler | 3 | 6 | low | 138 |

| Food | Carbo-hydrate g | Portion size | Fat g | Protein g | Fibre | kCalories per portion |
|---|---|---|---|---|---|---|
| **Strawberry jam** (conserve) | 10 | 1 level tbsp | 0 | trace | 0 | 39 |
| **Strawberry mousse** | 18 | 1 average serving | 6 | 4 | low | 137 |
| **Strawberry pavlova** | 45 | 1 average serving | 14 | 5 | med | 320 |
| **Strawberry shortcake** | 35 | 1 average serving | 12 | 5 | low | 265 |
| **Strawberry sorbet** | 19 | 1 scoop | trace | trace | low | 57 |
| **Strawberry soufflé** | 21 | 1 average serving | 41 | 6 | low | 325 |
| **Streusel cake** | 35 | 1 average slice | 1 | 3 | low | 157 |
| **Striped bass**, grilled (broiled) | 0 | 1 piece of fillet | 4 | 28 | 0 | 153 |
| **Stufato** (Italian beef stew) | 45 | 1 average serving | 16 | 6 | med | 565 |
| **Stuffing**, made with breadcrumbs and herbs | 3 | 1 level tbsp | trace | trace | low | 14 |
| Stuffing, made with rice | 5 | 1 level tbsp | 1 | trace | low | 31 |
| **Sugar puffs**, dry | 22 | 25 g/1 oz/½ cup | trace | 2 | low | 97 |
| Sugar puffs, with semi-skimmed milk | 41 | 5 heaped tbsp | 2 | 7 | low | 212 |
| Sugar puffs, with skimmed milk | 41 | 5 heaped tbsp | trace | 7 | low | 196 |
| **Sugar snap peas** | 8 | 10 pods | 1 | 5 | high | 57 |
| Sugar snap peas, steamed or boiled | 7 | 3 heaped tbsp | 1 | 5 | high | 52 |
| **Sugar**, all types | 5 | 1 level tsp | trace | trace | 0 | 20 |
| **Sukiyaki** | 20 | 1 average serving | 9 | 20 | high | 246 |
| **Sultana bran**, dry | 16 | 25 g/1 oz/½ cup | trace | 2 | high | 80 |

| Food | Carbo-hydrate g | Portion size | Fat g | Protein g | Fibre | kCalories per portion |
|------|------|------|------|------|------|------|
| Sultana bran, with semi-skimmed milk | 33 | 5 heaped tbsp | 3 | 8 | high | 185 |
| Sultana bran, with skimmed milk | 33 | 5 heaped tbsp | 1 | 8 | high | 169 |
| **Sultana (golden raisin) cake** | 29 | 1 average slice | 6 | 2 | med | 180 |
| **Sultanas** (golden raisins) | 10 | 1 small handful | trace | trace | high | 41 |
| **Summer pudding** | 59 | 1 average serving | 1 | 7 | high | 266 |
| **Sunflower seeds** | 2 | 1 level tbsp | 7 | 4 | high | 87 |
| **Supernoodles**, all flavours | 67 | 1 packet | 24 | 9 | high | 523 (average) |
| **Surf 'n' turf** | 17 | 1 steak plus 2 breaded prawns (shrimp) | 32 | 51 | low | 516 |
| **Sushi** | 8 | 1 piece | 1 | 1 | low | 40 |
| **Sussex pond pudding** | 50 | 1 average serving | 24 | 3 | low | 391 |
| **Sustain**, dry | 18 | 25 g/1 oz/½ cup | 1 | 2 | med | 90 |
| Sustain, with semi-skimmed milk | 36 | 5 heaped tbsp | 3 | 8 | med | 201 |
| Sustain, with skimmed milk | 36 | 5 heaped tbsp | 1 | 8 | med | 185 |
| **Swede** (rutabaga), steamed or boiled | 2 | 3 heaped tbsp | trace | trace | low | 11 |
| **Sweet and sour chicken** | 32 | 1 average serving | 2 | 6 | high | 165 |
| **Sweet and sour pork** | 31 | 1 average serving | 9 | 26 | med | 303 |
| **Sweet and sour sauce** | 16 | 5 level tbsp | trace | trace | low | 112 |

| Food | Carbo-hydrate g | Portion size | Fat g | Protein g | Fibre | kCalories per portion |
|---|---|---|---|---|---|---|
| **Sweet potatoes,** roasted | 20 | 4 pieces | 12 | 2 | med | 190 |
| Sweet potatoes, steamed or boiled, mashed | 20 | 3 heaped tbsp | trace | 1 | med | 84 |
| **Sweetcorn** (corn), kernels, canned | 27 | 3 heaped tbsp | 1 | 3 | med | 122 |
| Sweetcorn, on the cob *See also* Corn cobs *and* Corn on the cob | 17 | 1 cob | 2 | 4 | med | 99 |
| **Swiss chard,** steamed or boiled | 4 | 3 heaped tbsp | trace | 2 | med | 25 |
| **Swiss cheese** *See also* Emmental *and* Gruyère | 1 | 1 small wedge | 8 | 8 | 0 | 107 |
| **Swiss cheese fondue** | 8 | 1 average serving | 29 | 30 | 0 | 492 |
| Swiss cheese fondue, with French bread | 62 | 1 average serving plus 10 cubes of bread | 31 | 40 | med | 762 |
| **Swiss (jelly) roll,** chocolate | 14 | 1 individual roll | 3 | 3 | low | 85 |
| Swiss roll, with jam (conserve) | 24 | 1 individual roll | 1 | 1 | low | 105 |
| **Swiss-style muesli** *See* Muesli | | | | | | |
| **Swordfish steak,** fried (sautéed) | 0 | 1 medium steak | 14 | 44 | 0 | 294 |
| Swordfish steak, grilled (broiled) | 0 | 1 medium steak | 9 | 44 | 0 | 271 |

| Food | Carbo-hydrate g | Portion size | Fat g | Protein g | Fibre | kCalories per portion |
|------|-----------------|--------------|-------|-----------|-------|----------------------|
| **Syllabub** | 5 | 1 average serving | 35 | 1 | 0 | 428 |
| **Syrup, golden** (light corn) | 12 | 1 level tbsp | 0 | trace | 0 | 45 |
| **Syrup sauce**, for ice cream, bottled, all flavours | 23 | 2 level tbsp | 0 | trace | 0 | 92 (average) |
| **Syrup sponge pudding** | 53 | 1 average serving | 16 | 6 | med | 369 |
| **Syrup tart** | 60 | 1 average slice | 14 | 4 | med | 368 |

| Food | Carbo-hydrate g | Portion size | Fat g | Protein g | Fibre | kCalories per portion |
|---|---|---|---|---|---|---|
| **Tabbouleh** | **41** | 3 heaped tbsp | 10 | 7 | high | 278 |
| **Taco shell** | **6** | 1 shell | 3 | 1 | low | 57 |
| Taco shell, filled with chilli and salad | **12** | 1 shell | 10 | 7 | med | 170 |
| **Tagliarini** (pasta strands), dried, boiled | **51** | 1 average serving | 2 | 8 | med | 239 |
| Tagliarini, fresh, boiled | **57** | 1 average serving | 2 | 11 | med | 301 |
| **Tagliatelle** (pasta ribbons), dried, boiled | **51** | 1 average serving | 2 | 8 | med | 239 |
| Tagliatelle, fresh, boiled | **57** | 1 average serving | 2 | 11 | med | 301 |
| **Tahini paste** | **trace** | 1 level tbsp | 9 | 3 | med | 91 |
| **Tandoori chicken** | **7** | ½ small chicken | 38 | 95 | low | 750 |
| **Tangerine** | **11** | 1 fruit | trace | 1 | med | 44 |
| **Tangle twister** ice lolly | **18** | 1 lolly | 2 | 1 | low | 90 |
| **Tango**, lemon See also Apple tango, etc. | **23** | 1 tumbler | trace | trace | 0 | 98 |
| Tango, orange | **25** | 1 tumbler | 0 | 0 | 0 | 92 |
| **Tapioca pudding**, canned | **27** | ½ large can | 5 | 3 | low | 169 |
| Tapioca pudding, made with semi-skimmed milk | **29** | 1 average serving | 2 | 6 | low | 150 |
| Tapioca pudding, made with skimmed milk | **29** | 1 average serving | trace | 6 | low | 134 |

| Food | Carbo-hydrate g | Portion size | Fat g | Protein g | Fibre | kCalories per portion |
|------|------|------|------|------|------|------|
| **Taramasalata** | 2 | 2 level tbsp | 23 | 2 | low | 223 |
| **Tartare sauce** | 3 | 1 level tbsp | 3 | trace | low | 43 |
| **Taxi** chocolate bar | 17 | 1 standard bar | 7 | 1 | low | 134 |
| **Tea**, black | trace | 1 cup | trace | trace | 0 | 0 |
| Tea, with lemon | trace | 1 cup | trace | trace | 0 | 0 |
| Tea, with lemon and sugar | 5 | 1 cup plus 1 tsp of sugar | trace | trace | 0 | 20 |
| Tea, with milk | trace | 1 cup | 1 | trace | 0 | 7 |
| **Teacake** | 32 | 1 teacake | 4 | 5 | low | 180 |
| Teacake, toasted, with butter | 32 | 1 teacake | 12 | 5 | low | 254 |
| Teacake, toasted, with low-fat spread | 32 | 1 teacake | 8 | 6 | low | 219 |
| **Tempura** | 40 | 1 average serving | 8 | 23 | low | 328 |
| **Tequila** | trace | 1 single measure | 0 | trace | 0 | 55 |
| **Tequila sunrise** | 24 | 1 cocktail | trace | 1 | 0 | 232 |
| **Teriyaki sauce** | 3 | 1 level tbsp | trace | trace | low | 14 |
| **Thai chicken**, with noodles | 59 | 1 average serving | 15 | 34 | high | 506 |
| **Thai chicken soup** | 21 | 2 ladlefuls | 1 | 3 | low | 111 |
| **Thai fragrant rice**, steamed or boiled | 56 | 1 average serving | 2 | 5 | low | 248 |
| **Thousand island dressing** | 2 | 1 level tbsp | 5 | trace | low | 59 |
| Thousand island dressing, low-calorie | 1 | 1 level tbsp | 1 | trace | low | 12 |
| **Tia Maria** | 6 | 1 single measure | 0 | trace | 0 | 79 |

| Food | Carbo-hydrate g | Portion size | Fat g | Protein g | Fibre | kCalories per portion |
|---|---|---|---|---|---|---|
| Tilsit cheese | trace | 1 small wedge | 7 | 7 | 0 | 96 |
| Time out chocolate bar | 6 | 1 finger | 6 | 1 | low | 105 |
| Tip top topping | 1 | 1 level tbsp | 1 | 1 | low | 16 |
| Tipsy cake | 41 | 1 average slice | 32 | 5 | low | 488 |
| Tiramisu | 24 | 1 average serving | 11 | 6 | low | 222 |
| Tisanes, all flavours | trace | 1 cup | trace | trace | 0 | 0 |
| Tizer | 20 | 1 tumbler | trace | 0 | low | 82 |
| Tizer, diet | trace | 1 tumbler | trace | 0 | low | 0 |
| Toad-in-the-hole | 33 | 2 thick sausages plus batter | 30 | 17 | med | 462 |
| Toast, white, with butter | 18 | 1 medium slice | 9 | 3 | low | 155 |
| Toast, white, with low-fat spread | 18 | 1 medium slice | 5 | 4 | low | 120 |
| Toast, wholemeal, with butter | 15 | 1 medium slice | 10 | 3 | high | 153 |
| Toast, wholemeal, with low-fat spread | 15 | 1 medium slice | 6 | 4 | high | 118 |
| Toasted cheese and ham sandwiches | 36 | 1 round | 27 | 20 | med | 438 |
| Toffee bon bons | 6 | 1 toffee | 1 | 0 | 0 | 29 |
| Toffee apple | 66 | 1 apple | trace | 4 | high | 251 |
| Toffee crisp chocolate bar | 30 | 1 standard bar | 12 | 2 | low | 237 |
| Toffee fudge ice cream | 12 | 1 scoop | 4 | 1 | 0 | 90 |
| Toffees, mixed | 1 | 1 toffee | 0 | trace | 0 | 20 |
| Toffos, assorted | 31 | 1 tube | 8 | 1 | 0 | 203 |

| Food | Carbo-hydrate g | Portion size | Fat g | Protein g | Fibre | kCalories per portion |
|---|---|---|---|---|---|---|
| **Tofu**, firm | 2 | ½ block | 2 | 8 | low | 62 |
| Tofu, fried (sautéed) | 12 | ½ block | 24 | 20 | med | 308 |
| Tofu, marinated, baked | 4 | ½ block | 10 | 12 | med | 139 |
| Tofu, silken | 2 | ½ block | 2 | 5 | low | 55 |
| Tofu, smoked | 1 | ½ block | 9 | 36 | low | 148 |
| **Tofu and vegetable stir-fry** | 24 | 1 average serving | 21 | 17 | high | 334 |
| **Tofu burger** | 6 | 1 burger | 12 | 10 | med | 154 |
| **Tomato** | 2 | 1 fruit | trace | 1 | low | 13 |
| Tomato, stuffed, baked | 9 | 1 large tomato | 1 | 3 | med | 53 |
| **Tomato and herb pasta sauce**, ready-made | 16 | ¼ jar | trace | 1 | low | 79 |
| **Tomato and lentil soup**, canned | 20 | 2 ladlefuls | trace | 6 | med | 108 |
| Tomato and lentil soup, home-made | 26 | 2 ladlefuls | 8 | 8 | med | 188 |
| Tomato and lentil soup, instant | 15 | 1 mug | 1 | 3 | low | 73 |
| **Tomato and onion salad** | 11 | 1 average serving | trace | 2 | med | 35 |
| Tomato and onion salad, dressed | 11 | 1 average serving | 17 | 2 | med | 132 |
| **Tomato and orange soup**, canned | 17 | 2 ladlefuls | 1 | 2 | low | 80 |
| Tomato and orange soup, home-made | 15 | 2 ladlefuls | 4 | 2 | med | 103 |

| Food | Carbo-hydrate g | Portion size | Fat g | Protein g | Fibre | kCalories per portion |
|---|---|---|---|---|---|---|
| **Tomato and rice soup**, canned | 17 | 2 ladlefuls | 2 | 2 | low | 94 |
| **Tomato chutney** | 6 | 1 level tbsp | trace | trace | low | 24 |
| **Tomato juice** | 6 | 1 tumbler | trace | 2 | med | 28 |
| **Tomato juice cocktail** | 19 | 1 tumbler | 0 | 2 | low | 36 |
| **Tomato ketchup** (catsup) | 4 | 1 level tbsp | trace | trace | low | 15 |
| **Tomato relish** | 3 | 1 level tbsp | trace | trace | low | 16 |
| **Tomato risotto** | 58 | 1 average serving | 18 | 7 | med | 403 |
| **Tomato sauce**, home-made | 6 | 5 level tbsp | 4 | 2 | med | 67 |
| **Tomato soup**, cream of, canned | 12 | 2 ladlefuls | 7 | 2 | low | 110 |
| Tomato soup, home-made | 11 | 2 ladlefuls | 4 | 3 | low | 86 |
| Tomato soup, instant | 17 | 1 mug | 2 | 1 | med | 85 |
| Tomato soup, low-fat, canned | 8 | 2 ladlefuls | 1 | 1 | low | 50 |
| **Tomatoes**, canned | 6 | 1 small can | trace | 2 | med | 32 |
| Tomatoes, fried (sautéed) | 4 | 2 halves | 6 | trace | low | 68 |
| Tomatoes, grilled (broiled) | 7 | 2 halves | 1 | 1 | low | 37 |
| Tomatoes, sieved | 6 | 5 tbsp | trace | 1 | 0 | 29 |
| Tomatoes, stewed | 4 | 2 whole | trace | 1 | med | 25 |
| Tomatoes, sun-dried | 1 | 1 piece | trace | trace | low | 5 |
| Tomatoes, sun-dried, in oil, drained | 1 | 1 piece | 1 | trace | low | 7 |

| Food | Carbo-hydrate g | Portion size | Fat g | Protein g | Fibre | kCalories per portion |
|---|---|---|---|---|---|---|
| **Tongue**, lunch | 0 | 1 medium slice | 3 | 1 | 0 | 43 |
| Tongue, ox, pressed and sliced | 0 | 1 medium slice | 6 | 5 | 0 | 73 |
| Tongue, pork, pressed and sliced | 0 | 1 medium slice | 4 | 1 | 0 | 47 |
| **Tongues**, lambs', canned | 0 | ½ medium can | 16 | 16 | 0 | 213 |
| **Tonic water** | 10 | 1 tumbler | 0 | 0 | 0 | 43 |
| Tonic water, low-calorie | 0 | 1 tumbler | 0 | trace | 0 | 4 |
| **Topic** chocolate bar | 27 | 1 standard bar | 12 | 3 | low | 233 |
| **Tornado** ice cream | 15 | 1 ice | 0 | 0 | 0 | 61 |
| **Tortellini** (stuffed pasta), dried, boiled | 45 | 1 average serving | 6 | 9 | med | 291 |
| Tortellini, fresh, boiled | 40 | 1 average serving | 4 | 9 | med | 229 |
| **Tortilla** (Spanish omelette) | 17 | 2 eggs | 22 | 16 | med | 328 |
| **Tortilla chips**, all flavours | 30 | 1 small bag | 11 | 4 | med | 229 |
| **Tortillas**, corn | 12 | 1 medium tortilla | 1 | 1 | med | 58 |
| Tortillas, flour | 27 | 1 medium tortilla | 3 | 4 | med | 159 |
| **Tournedos rossini** | 9 | 1 medium steak | 25 | 52 | low | 477 |
| **Tracker bars**, all flavours | 22 | 1 standard bar | 10 | 3 | med | 192 (average) |
| **Treacle**, black (molasses) | 10 | 1 level tbsp | 0 | trace | 0 | 38 |
| **Treacle pudding** | 53 | 1 average serving | 16 | 6 | med | 369 |
| **Treacle tart** | 60 | 1 slice | 14 | 4 | med | 368 |
| **Treacle toffee** | 1 | 1 piece | 0 | trace | 0 | 20 |

| Food | Carbo-hydrate g | Portion size | Fat g | Protein g | Fibre | kCalories per portion |
|---|---|---|---|---|---|---|
| Trifle | 69 | 1 average serving | 6 | 10 | high | 372 |
| Trinity cream | 15 | 1 average serving | 50 | 1 | 0 | 453 |
| Trio chocolate bar | 12 | 1 standard bar | 6 | 1 | low | 111 |
| Triple chocolate bar | 12 | 1 standard bar | 5 | 1 | low | 99 |
| Tropical fruit salad | 22 | 3 heaped tbsp | trace | trace | med | 86 |
| Trout, baked, stuffed | 41 | 1 medium fish | 39 | 56 | med | 726 |
| Trout, fried (sautéed) | 0 | 1 medium fish | 13 | 33 | 0 | 232 |
| Trout, grilled (broiled) | 0 | 1 medium fish | 8 | 33 | 0 | 209 |
| Trout, poached or steamed | 0 | 1 medium fish | 7 | 35 | 0 | 200 |
| Trout, smoked | 0 | 1 medium fillet | 5 | 23 | 0 | 136 |
| Trout, smoked, pâté | 0 | 1 average serving | 24 | 11 | 0 | 269 |
| Trout meunière | trace | 1 medium fish | 29 | 46 | 0 | 388 |
| Trout with almonds | 1 | 1 med fish | 36 | 48 | med | 464 |
| Truffles | 6 | 1 truffle | 2 | 1 | low | 50 |
| Truite au bleu | 0 | 1 medium fish | 7 | 35 | 0 | 200 |
| Tuc crackers | 3 | 1 cracker | 1 | trace | low | 25 |
| Tuc savoury sandwiches | 7 | 1 sandwich | 5 | 1 | low | 76 |
| Tuna, canned in brine, drained | 0 | ½ standard can | trace | 23 | 0 | 107 |
| Tuna, canned in oil, drained | 0 | ½ standard can | 7 | 27 | 0 | 182 |
| Tuna and cucumber sandwiches | 35 | 1 round | 18 | 15 | med | 352 |
| Tuna and pasta casserole | 30 | 1 average serving | 9 | 22 | med | 285 |

| Food | Carbo-hydrate g | Portion size | Fat g | Protein g | Fibre | kCalories per portion |
|---|---|---|---|---|---|---|
| **Tuna and sweetcorn pasta** | 50 | 1 average serving | 11 | 37 | med | 451 |
| **Tuna mornay** | 7 | 1 average serving | 10 | 29 | low | 241 |
| **Tuna mousse** | 6 | 1 average serving | 10 | 11 | low | 185 |
| **Tuna salad** | 5 | 1 average serving | 1 | 25 | high | 138 |
| Tuna salad, with mayonnaise | 11 | 1 average serving | 23 | 25 | high | 344 |
| **Tuna steak**, fried (sautéed) | 0 | 1 medium steak | 15 | 52 | 0 | 345 |
| Tuna steak, grilled (broiled) | 0 | 1 medium steak | 10 | 52 | 0 | 322 |
| **Tunes** sweets (candies) | 36 | 1 tube | 0 | 0 | 0 | 145 |
| **Turbot**, grilled (broiled) | 0 | 1 piece of fillet | 6 | 33 | 0 | 194 |
| Turbot, steamed or poached | 0 | 1 piece of fillet | 1 | 36 | 0 | 159 |
| **Turkey**, breast, smoked | trace | 1 medium slice | trace | 4 | 0 | 21 |
| Turkey, fillets, fried (sautéed) | 0 | 1 medium fillet | 9 | 40 | 0 | 248 |
| Turkey fillets, grilled (broiled) | 0 | 1 medium fillet | 4 | 40 | 0 | 225 |
| Turkey fillets, fried, in breadcrumbs | 13 | 1 medium fillet | 9 | 43 | low | 326 |
| Turkey, minced (ground), stewed | 0 | 1 average serving | 5 | 31 | 0 | 197 |
| Turkey, roast, with skin | 0 | 2 medium slices | 6 | 28 | 0 | 171 |
| Turkey, roast, without skin | 0 | 2 medium slices | 3 | 29 | 0 | 140 |

| Food | Carbo-hydrate g | Portion size | Fat g | Protein g | Fibre | kCalories per portion |
|---|---|---|---|---|---|---|
| Turkey, roast, with stuffing and sausagemeat | 12 | 1 average serving | 5 | 33 | med | 229 |
| Turkey and vegetable casserole | 32 | 1 average serving | 8 | 23 | med | 298 |
| Turkey and vegetable soup, home-made | 14 | 2 ladlefuls | 4 | 10 | med | 134 |
| Turkey and vegetable stir-fry | 31 | 1 average serving | 3 | 29 | high | 259 |
| Turkey bacon, grilled (broiled) | trace | 1 med slice | 3 | 2 | 0 | 34 |
| Turkey burger in a bun, with relish, home-made | 32 | 1 burger in a bun | 9 | 38 | low | 357 |
| Turkey fingers, fried (sautéed), in batter or breadcrumbs | 11 | 1 finger | 11 | 9 | low | 178 |
| Turkey ham | trace | 1 med slice | 1 | 5 | 0 | 36 |
| Turkey pot pie | 28 | 1 average slice | 39 | 17 | low | 485 |
| Turkey roll | trace | 1 med slice | 2 | 5 | 0 | 41 |
| Turkey sandwiches | 34 | 1 round | 19 | 10 | med | 345 |
| Turkey soup, home-made | 7 | 2 ladlefuls | 2 | 13 | 0 | 111 |
| Turkey stew | 65 | 1 average serving | 3 | 34 | med | 430 |
| Turkish delight, chocolate covered | 37 | 1 standard bar | 4 | 1 | 0 | 185 |

| Food | Carbo-hydrate g | Portion size | Fat g | Protein g | Fibre | kCalories per portion |
|---|---|---|---|---|---|---|
| Turkish delight, in icing (confectioners') sugar | 8 | 1 cube | 0 | trace | 0 | 29 |
| Turnips, glazed | 15 | 3 heaped tbsp | trace | 1 | med | 55 |
| Turnips, steamed or boiled | 2 | 3 heaped tbsp | trace | 1 | med | 12 |
| Tuscan bean salad | 12 | 3 heaped tbsp | 5 | 4 | high | 120 |
| Tutti frutti ice cream | 5 | 1 scoop | 7 | 1 | low | 75 |
| Twiglets | 16 | 1 small bag | 3 | 4 | med | 136 |
| Twirl chocolate bar | 12 | 1 finger | 7 | 2 | 0 | 115 |
| Twistetti (pasta shapes), dried, boiled | 42 | 1 average serving | 1 | 7 | med | 198 |
| Twistetti, fresh, boiled | 45 | 1 average serving | 2 | 9 | med | 235 |
| Twix chocolate bar | 18 | 1 finger | 7 | 2 | low | 143 |
| Twix ice cream | 23 | 1 standard bar | 14 | 3 | low | 228 |
| Tzatziki | 1 | 2 level tbsp | 1 | 1 | low | 20 |

| Food | Carbo-hydrate g | Portion size | Fat g | Protein g | Fibre | kCalories per portion |
|---|---|---|---|---|---|---|
| **Vacherin**, with cream and fruit | 45 | 1 average slice | 14 | 5 | med | 320 |
| **Vanilla fudge** | 14 | 1 square | 2 | trace | 0 | 77 |
| **Vanilla cheesecake** | 30 | 1 average slice | 27 | 4 | low | 490 |
| **Vanilla ice cream,** dairy | 12 | 1 scoop | 5 | 2 | 0 | 97 |
| Vanilla ice cream, non-dairy | 11 | 1 scoop | 4 | 2 | 0 | 89 |
| **Vanilla soufflé** | 26 | 1 average serving | 1 | 7 | low | 236 |
| **Veal, cutlet**, fried (sautéed), in breadcrumbs, | 8 | 1 cutlet | 14 | 55 | low | 376 |
| Veal, cutlet, grilled (broiled) | 0 | 1 cutlet | 9 | 52 | 0 | 300 |
| Veal, escalope, fried, in breadcrumbs | 20 | 1 escalope | 15 | 32 | low | 335 |
| Veal, roast | 0 | 2 thick slices | 11 | 32 | 0 | 230 |
| **Veal birds** | 12 | 2 rolls | 20 | 52 | low | 450 |
| **Veal fricassée** | 34 | 1 average serving | 9 | 27 | low | 339 |
| **Vegemite** | trace | 1 level tsp | 0 | 1 | 0 | 8 |
| **Vegetable bake** | 33 | 1 average serving | 10 | 12 | high | 360 |
| **Vegetable casserole** | 33 | 1 average serving | 6 | 12 | high | 228 |
| **Vegetable cottage pie** | 48 | 1 average serving | 12 | 15 | high | 350 |
| **Vegetable curry** | 34 | 1 average serving | 4 | 5 | high | 183 |
| **Vegetable deluxe burger** | 54 | 1 burger in a bun | 18 | 10 | high | 423 |
| **Vegetable goulash** | 142 | 1 average serving | 15 | 12 | high | 338 |
| **Vegetable juice** | 9 | 1 tumbler | trace | trace | 0 | 41 |

| Food | Carbo-hydrate g | Portion size | Fat g | Protein g | Fibre | kCalories per portion |
|---|---|---|---|---|---|---|
| **Vegetable lasagne** | **50** | 1 average serving | 10 | 15 | high | 424 |
| **Vegetable pâté** | **1** | 1 average serving | 10 | 10 | low | 138 |
| **Vegetable pie** | **52** | 1 individual pie | 23 | 6 | med | 425 |
| **Vegetable risotto** | **58** | 1 average serving | 15 | 6 | low | 372 |
| **Vegetable samosa** | **11** | 1 samosa | 21 | 1 | med | 236 |
| **Vegetable soup,** canned | **13** | 2 ladlefuls | 1 | 3 | high | 74 |
| Vegetable soup, home-made | **4** | 2 ladlefuls | trace | 3 | high | 93 |
| Vegetable soup, packet | **8** | 2 ladlefuls | 1 | 2 | low | 46 |
| **Vegetable stew** | **31** | 1 average serving | 4 | 7 | high | 186 |
| **Vegetable stir-fry** | **15** | 1 average serving | 6 | 7 | high | 169 |
| **Vegetable terrine** | **17** | 1 thick slice | 7 | 8 | high | 155 |
| **Vegetables**, mixed, canned, drained | **6** | 3 heaped tbsp | 1 | 2 | med | 38 |
| Vegetables, mixed, frozen, cooked | **7** | 3 heaped tbsp | trace | 3 | high | 42 |
| **Veggie burger** | **5** | 1 burger | 4 | 7 | med | 85 |
| **Veggie sausage** | **6** | 1 sausage | 4 | 3 | med | 75 |
| **Velouté sauce** | **4** | 5 level tbsp | 9 | 1 | low | 99 |
| **Venison**, roast | **0** | 2 thick slices | 6 | 35 | 0 | 198 |
| Venison, stewed | **0** | 1 average serving | 7 | 25 | 0 | 225 |
| **Vermicelli** (pasta strands), dried, boiled | **51** | 1 average serving | 2 | 8 | med | 239 |
| Vermicelli, fresh, boiled | **57** | 1 average serving | 2 | 11 | med | 301 |
| **Vermouth**, bianco | **8** | 1 double measure | 0 | trace | 0 | 67 |

| Food | Carbo-hydrate g | Portion size | Fat g | Protein g | Fibre | kCalories per portion |
|---|---|---|---|---|---|---|
| Vermouth, extra dry | 3 | 1 double measure | 0 | trace | 0 | 59 |
| Vermouth, red | 8 | 1 double measure | 0 | trace | 0 | 75 |
| Vermouth, rosso | 8 | 1 double measure | 0 | trace | 0 | 85 |
| **Vichyssoise**, canned | 12 | 2 ladlefuls | 6 | 2 | low | 108 |
| Vichyssoise, home-made | 8 | 2 ladlefuls | 6 | 2 | low | 117 |
| **Victoria sandwich**, filled with jam (conserve) | 64 | 1 average slice | 5 | 4 | low | **302** |
| **Viennetta**, all flavours | 23 | 1 average slice | 14 | 3 | 0 | 227 (average) |
| **Vienna bread** | 15 | 1 thick slice | 1 | 3 | low | 109 |
| **Viennese finger**, filled | 9 | 1 biscuit (cookie) | 5 | 1 | low | 81 |
| **Vimto** | 20 | 1 tumbler | trace | trace | 0 | 52 |
| **Vinaigrette dressing** | trace | 1 tbsp | 11 | trace | 0 | 101 |
| Vinaigrette dressing, low-calorie | 1 | 1 tbsp | trace | trace | 0 | 5 |
| **Vine leaves**, stuffed | 19 | 2 rolls | 9 | 18 | high | 221 |
| **Vinegar**, all types | 0 | 1 tsp | 0 | trace | 0 | 1 |
| **Vitbe bread** | 16 | 1 med slice | 1 | 3 | med | 82 |
| **Vitello tonnato** | 20 | 1 escalope | 37 | 44 | low | 594 |
| **Vodka** | trace | 1 single measure | 0 | trace | 0 | 55 |
| Vodka and orange | 7 | 1 single measure | 0 | trace | 0 | 108 |
| Vodka and tonic | 5 | 1 single measure plus 1 mixer | 0 | trace | 0 | 76 |
| Vodka and tonic, low-calorie | trace | 1 single measure plus 1 mixer | trace | trace | 0 | 58 |

| Food | Carbo-hydrate g | Portion size | Fat g | Protein g | Fibre | kCalories per portion |
|------|------|------|------|------|------|------|
| **Vodka martini** | **3** | 1 cocktail | trace | trace | 0 | 114 |
| **Vol-au-vents**, all flavours | **20** | 1 med | 18 | 11 | low | 286 (average) |
| Vol-au-vents, cocktail, all flavours | 10 | 1 small | 9 | 5 | low | 143 (average) |

| Food | Carbo-hydrate g | Portion size | Fat g | Protein g | Fibre | kCalories per portion |
|---|---|---|---|---|---|---|
| **Wafer biscuits** (cookies), chocolate-covered | **13** | 1 biscuit | 6 | 1 | low | 115 |
| Wafer biscuits, filled | **7** | 1 biscuit | 2 | 1 | low | 39 |
| **Wafers**, for ice cream | **4** | 1 wafer | trace | 2 | low | 17 |
| **Waffle**, potato, fried (sautéed) or baked | **13** | 1 waffle | 3 | 1 | low | 84 |
| Waffle, sweet | **30** | 1 waffle | 8 | 8 | low | 240 |
| Waffles, sweet, with maple syrup | **75** | 2 waffles | 16 | 16 | med | 533 |
| Waffles, with bacon and maple syrup | **75** | 2 waffles plus 2 rashers (slices) of bacon | 48 | 36 | med | 799 |
| **Walnut cake** | **34** | 1 average slice | 19 | 7 | med | 344 |
| **Walnut whip** | **20** | 1 whip | 8 | 7 | low | 165 |
| **Walnut whirl**, chocolate | **2** | 1 chocolate | 1 | trace | low | 20 |
| **Walnuts**, shelled | **1** | 25 g/1 oz/¼ cup | 17 | 4 | high | 172 |
| **Water biscuits** (crackers) | **6** | 1 biscuit | 1 | 1 | low | 33 |
| **Water chestnuts**, canned, drained | **3** | 4 pieces | trace | trace | low | 14 |
| **Watercress** | **trace** | 1 good handful | trace | trace | med | 3 |
| **Watercress soup** | **14** | 2 ladlefuls | 2 | 1 | low | 99 |
| **Watermelon** | **14** | 1 large wedge | 1 | 1 | low | 66 |
| **Weetabix**, dry | **13** | 1 biscuit | trace | 2 | high | 64 |
| Weetabix, with semi-skimmed milk | **32** | 2 biscuits | trace | 8 | high | 169 |

| Food | Carbo-hydrate g | Portion size | Fat g | Protein g | Fibre | kCalories per portion |
|---|---|---|---|---|---|---|
| Weetabix, with skimmed milk | **32** | 2 biscuits | 2 | 8 | high | 185 |
| **Weetaflakes**, dry | 20 | 25 g/1 oz/½ cup | 1 | 2 | high | 90 |
| Weetaflakes, with semi-skimmed milk | **38** | 5 heaped tbsp | 3 | 8 | high | 201 |
| Weetaflakes, with skimmed milk | **38** | 5 heaped tbsp | 1 | 8 | high | 185 |
| **Weetos**, dry | 20 | 25 g/1 oz/½ cup | 1 | 1 | med | 96 |
| Weetos, with semi-skimmed milk | **30** | 5 heaped tbsp | 4 | 6 | med | 172 |
| Weetos, with skimmed milk | **30** | 5 heaped tbsp | 2 | 6 | med | 154 |
| **Welsh rarebit** | 21 | 1 medium slice | 13 | 10 | low | 242 |
| **Wensleydale cheese** | trace | 1 small wedge | 8 | 6 | 0 | 94 |
| **Westphalian ham** | trace | 1 thin slice | 2 | 4 | 0 | 29 |
| **Wheat bran** | 4 | 1 level tbsp | 1 | 2 | high | 31 |
| **Wheat crunchies**, all flavours | 20 | 1 small packet | 9 | 4 | low | 180 (average) |
| **Whelks**, boiled | trace | 1 average serving | trace | 3 | 0 | 14 |
| **Whippy ice cream** | 12 | 1 cornet | 3 | 2 | low | 85 |
| **Whisky** | trace | 1 single measure | 0 | trace | 0 | 55 |
| **Whisky and coke** | 6 | 1 single measure plus 1 mixer | 0 | trace | 0 | 99 |
| **Whisky and coke, low-calorie** | trace | 1 single measure plus 1 mixer | trace | trace | 0 | 56 |
| **Whisky and ginger ale** | 5 | 1 single measure plus 1 mixer | 0 | trace | 0 | 75 |
| Whisky and ginger ale, low-calorie | trace | 1 single measure plus 1 tumbler | 0 | trace | 0 | 55 |

| Food | Carbo-hydrate g | Portion size | Fat g | Protein g | Fibre | kCalories per portion |
|---|---|---|---|---|---|---|
| **Whisky mac** | trace | 1 single measure plus 1 double measure | 0 | trace | 0 | 255 |
| **Whisky sour** | 14 | 1 cocktail | 0 | 0 | 0 | 157 |
| **White pudding,** fried (sautéed) or baked | 36 | 2 thick slices | 32 | 7 | low | 450 |
| **White sauce,** savoury, made with semi-skimmed milk | 8 | 5 level tbsp | 6 | 3 | low | 96 |
| White sauce, savoury, made with skimmed milk | 8 | 5 level tbsp | 5 | 3 | low | 86 |
| White sauce, sweet, made with semi-skimmed milk | 14 | 5 level tbsp | 5 | 3 | low | 112 |
| White sauce, sweet, made with skimmed milk | 14 | 5 level tbsp | 4 | 3 | low | 92 |
| **White Stilton cheese** | trace | 1 small wedge | 8 | 6 | 0 | 94 |
| **White wine sauce** | 6 | 5 level tbsp | 2 | 2 | low | 75 |
| **Whitebait,** fried (sautéed) | 5 | 1 average serving | 47 | 19 | low | 525 |
| **Whiting,** fried (sautéed), in breadcrumbs | 12 | 1 medium fillet | 17 | 31 | low | 334 |
| Whiting, poached or steamed | 0 | 1 medium fillet | 1 | 24 | 0 | 110 |
| Whiting, smoked, poached | 1 | 1 medium fillet | 1 | 25 | 0 | 166 |

| Food | Carbo-hydrate g | Portion size | Fat g | Protein g | Fibre | kCalories per portion |
|------|------|------|------|------|------|------|
| **Wholegrain mustard** | 1 | 1 level tsp | trace | 2 | low | 7 |
| **Wholenut** chocolate bar | 24 | 1 standard bar | 17 | 5 | med | 270 |
| **Whopper** | 47 | 1 burger | 40 | 29 | high | 660 |
| Whopper, with cheese | 47 | 1 burger | 48 | 35 | high | 760 |
| Whopper, double | 47 | 2 burgers | 21 | 49 | high | 920 |
| Whopper, double, with cheese | 47 | 2 burgers | 67 | 55 | high | 1010 |
| **Wiener schnitzel** | 20 | 1 schnitzel | 15 | 32 | low | 335 |
| **Wild rice**, cooked | 6 | 1 average serving | trace | 7 | 0 | 182 |
| **Wild rice mix**, cooked | 31 | 1 average serving | 1 | 6 | low | 177 |
| **Winders**, real fruit | 11 | 1 roll | 1 | trace | low | 55 |
| **Wine gums** | 27 | 1 tube | trace | 3 | 0 | 119 |
| **Wine**, dry white | 1 | 1 wine glass | 0 | trace | 0 | 82 |
| Wine, dry white, sparkling | 2 | 1 wine glass | 0 | trace | 0 | 95 |
| Wine, low-alcohol, red | 2 | 1 wine glass | 0 | trace | 0 | 70 |
| Wine, low-alcohol, rosé | 2 | 1 wine glass | 0 | trace | 0 | 70 |
| Wine, low-alcohol, white | 2 | 1 wine glass | 0 | trace | 0 | 70 |
| Wine, medium white | 4 | 1 wine glass | 0 | trace | 0 | 94 |
| Wine, mulled | 5 | 1 wine glass | 0 | trace | 0 | 105 |
| Wine, red | **trace** | 1 wine glass | trace | trace | 0 | 85 |
| Wine, rosé | 1 | 1 wine glass | 0 | trace | 0 | 89 |

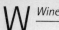 

| Food | Carbo-hydrate g | Portion size | Fat g | Protein g | Fibre | kCalories per portion |
|---|---|---|---|---|---|---|
| Wine, sweet | 7 | 1 wine glass | 0 | trace | 0 | 117 |
| Winkles | trace | 1 average serving | trace | 3 | 0 | 14 |
| Winter radish | 2 | 1 radish | trace | 1 | low | 12 |
| Wispa chocolate bar | 21 | 1 standard bar | 13 | 3 | 0 | 210 |
| Wispa, gold | 29 | 1 standard bar | 15 | 3 | 0 | 265 |
| Wispa, mint | 27 | 1 standard bar | 17 | 3 | 0 | 275 |
| Witch, fried (sautéed), in breadcrumbs | 15 | 1 medium fish | 21 | 25 | low | 342 |
| Witch, grilled (broiled) | 0 | 1 medium fish | 4 | 25 | 0 | 158 |
| Witch, poached or steamed | 0 | 1 medium fish | 1 | 25 | 0 | 112 |
| Woodcock, roast | 0 | 1 bird | 18 | 37 | 0 | 303 |
| Worcestershire sauce | 4 | 1 tbsp | 0 | trace | 0 | 17 |
| Wotsits, all flavours | 12 | 1 small packet | 7 | 2 | low | 115 (average) |

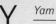 

| Food | Carbo-hydrate g | Portion size | Fat g | Protein g | Fibre | kCalories per portion |
|------|------|------|------|------|------|------|
| **Yam**, roast | **33** | 4 pieces | 5 | 2 | med | 156 |
| Yam, steamed or boiled, mashed | **33** | 3 heaped tbsp | trace | 2 | med | 133 |
| **Yeast extract** | **trace** | 1 level tsp | trace | 2 | 0 | 9 |
| **Yellow bean sauce** | **4** | 1 level tbsp | trace | trace | low | 19 |
| **Yellow beans**, fresh, steamed or boiled | **5** | 3 heaped tbsp | trace | 2 | high | 25 |
| **Yellow melon** | **15** | 1 large wedge | trace | 1 | med | 63 |
| **Yoghurt** (plain) | **10** | 1 individual pot | 4 | 7 | 0 | 99 |
| Yoghurt, all flavours | **20** | 1 individual pot | 4 | 6 | 0 | 131 (average) |
| Yoghurt, bio | **7** | 1 small pot | 1 | 5 | 0 | 56 |
| Yoghurt, custard-style | **3** | 1 small pot | 13 | 8 | 0 | 161 |
| Yoghurt, drinking | **26** | 1 tumbler | trace | 6 | 0 | 124 |
| Yoghurt, fruit corner | **26** | 1 carton | 7 | 6 | low | 219 |
| Yoghurt, Greek-style, cows' | **3** | 1 individual pot | 13 | 8 | 0 | 161 |
| Yoghurt, Greek-style, sheep's | **8** | 1 individual pot | 10 | 6 | 0 | 149 |
| Yoghurt, low-calorie, plain | **7** | 1 individual pot | trace | 5 | 0 | 51 |
| Yoghurt, low-fat, plain | **9** | 1 individual pot | 1 | 6 | 0 | 70 |
| Yoghurt, low-fat, all flavours | **22** | 1 individual pot | 1 | 5 | 0 | 112 (average) |
| Yoghurt, soya | **5** | 1 individual pot | 5 | 6 | 0 | 90 |
| **Yoghurt ice-cream**, all flavours | **8** | 1 scoop | 1 | 3 | low | 53 (average) |

| Food | Carbo-hydrate g | Portion size | Fat g | Protein g | Fibre | kCalories per portion |
|------|------|------|------|------|------|------|
| **Yoghurt jelly** (jello), made with plain, low-fat yoghurt | 12 | 1 average serving | 1 | 5 | 0 | 60 |
| **Yorkie bar**, milk | 35 | 1 standard bar | 18 | 4 | 0 | 317 |
| Yorkie bar, nut | 26 | 1 standard bar | 10 | 6 | low | 312 |
| Yorkie bar, raisin and biscuit (cookie) | 32 | 1 standard bar | 13 | 3 | low | 265 |
| **Yorkshire parkin** | 29 | 1 average piece | 7 | 2 | low | 185 |
| **Yorkshire pudding** | 7 | 1 small pudding | 3 | 2 | low | 62 |

| Food | Carbo-hydrate g | Portion size | Fat g | Protein g | Fibre | kCalories per portion |
|---|---|---|---|---|---|---|
| **Zabaglione** | 8 | 1 average serving | 3 | 3 | 0 | 87 |
| **Zite** (pasta shapes), dried, boiled | 42 | 1 average serving | 1 | 7 | med | 198 |
| Zite, fresh, boiled | 45 | 1 average serving | 2 | 9 | med | 235 |
| **Zoom** ice lolly | 10 | 1 lolly | trace | trace | 0 | 46 |
| **Zucchini** See Courgettes | | | | | | |